Aromatherapy

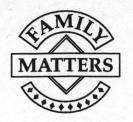

Aromatherapy

JULIE SADLER

WARD LOCK

A WARD LOCK BOOK

This edition published in the UK in 1994 by Ward Lock
Villiers House, 41/47 Strand, London WC2N 5JE

A Cassell Imprint

Distributed in the United States
by Sterling Publishing Co., Inc.
387 Park Avenue South, New York, NY 10016-8810

Distributed in Australia
by Capricorn Link (Australia) Pty Ltd
2/13 Carrington Road, Castle Hill, NSW 2154

British Library Cataloguing-in-Publication Data
A catalogue record for this book is available from the British Library

ISBN 0-7063-7227-1

Typeset by Columns of Reading

Printed and bound in Great Britain

Cover photograph: Larry Dale Gordon/Image Bank.

CONTENTS

Chapter 1

UNDERSTANDING AROMATHERAPY

Aromatherapy is a wonderful way of experiencing the many benefits of essential oils, but you may wonder what these little magic oils are. They are substances extracted from the roots, stalks, flowers, leaves or fruit of a plant and have numerous and powerful healing properties. Essential oils are also known as aromatherapy oils, so don't be confused if you are looking for one and can only find the other — they are the same thing!

I know from several years' experience of treating people just like you or I how the stresses and strains brought about by our hectic lifestyles can have a detrimental effect on our well-being.

Fortunately, this is where aromatherapy can come to the rescue! Everyone from a tiny baby to Grandma can enjoy the gentle aromatherapy experience.

AN ANCIENT CONCEPT IN A MODERN AGE

The roots of aromatherapy can be traced back to the early Egyptian empire 5,000 years ago. Clay tablets used to order the essential oils of myrrh and cypress, dating from about 1800 BC, were found in Babylon. So although no one is quite certain how or when aromatherapy originated it is definitely not a recent discovery.

There is a lot of evidence to suggest the ancient Egyptians used essential oils for embalming their dead. All the oils have antiseptic properties and would have greatly slowed down the decomposition of the body. The Egyptians passed on their knowledge to the ancient Greeks, who took to using essential oils in their medical treatments.

The Romans used essential oils more lavishly to beautify themselves. They would rub them into their skins both before and after bathing, and use them to perfume their clothes and hair. Eventually the Romans brought their knowledge to Britain. During the Great Plague of the Middle Ages people wore pomanders impregnated with essential oils, churches were fumigated with frankincense and pepper, and incense was continually burned in houses. Aromatic substances were used everywhere as they were the most effective antiseptic available at that time. Glove makers supposedly escaped the Black Death because they were protected by the essential oils they used to perfume gloves. Also, up until the nineteenth century physicians would carry little containers filled with essential oils on their walking canes, believing these would protect them from contagious diseases. Sadly, during the nineteenth century, essences began to be copied chemically to lower their cost. This resulted in the loss of their therapeutic properties.

In the early twentieth century, research began in earnest once again. One important figure was the French scientist René Maurice Gattefosse, who discovered for himself just how healing essential oils can be. He badly burned his hand and quickly immersed it in lavender essential oil, the nearest available cool liquid. Amazed at how quickly the burn healed, with no sign of a scar, he continued to research the oils much further and also coined the term aromatherapy. During the First World War he experimented with essential oils on soldiers' wounds, and found that they accelerated the healing process. He continued to research into the healing powers of essential oils and classified their effects on the human nervous system, metabolism, vital organs and endocrine system.

AROMATHERAPY AT HOME

Regular use of aromatherapy is a gentle, effective way of maintaining good health. In old Eastern medicine people visited their physicians in order to stay well, believing in the old adage 'Prevention is better than cure.'

Today we can help our bodies to function more efficiently, and alleviate the effects of stress and tension, by using aromatherapy in a number of different ways. Most of the treatments are simple enough for anyone to try at home.

BATHING

An aromatherapy bath is a lovely way to round off a tiring, stressful day. When essential oils are added to water they stimulate the skin and have a muscle-relaxing effect.

If you choose an uplifting oil an aromatherapy bath can be a great pick-me-up. I find lemon essential oil mixed with peppermint is good for this and helps soothe aching feet.

Aromatherapy baths can help:
☆ Nervous tension
☆ Headache
☆ Fatigue
☆ Muscular aches and pains

☆ Colds and flu
☆ Period pains

STEAMING AND INHALATION

Some conditions respond extremely well to essential oil inhalation. I'm sure we've all tried putting our heads over a bowl of steaming water mixed with friar's balsam to try to clear a stuffy nose. Well, we can use aromatherapy in the same way. There are many different oils to choose from and all of them are relieving and pleasant.

Steaming with essential oils can also be used to deep-cleanse and moisten the face, helping to maintain a healthy, supple skin. The oils can also be inhaled from a handkerchief or tissue; very useful for carrying around to relieve a cold or headache. You can also try a few drops on your pillow: it's marvellous how this can give enough relief to allow you a decent night's sleep.

COMPRESSES

Aromatherapy compresses can be helpful in the treatment of:
☆ Bruises
☆ Muscular aches and pains
☆ Irritated skin conditions
Usually you would soak the compress in approximately ½ pint (300 ml) of water to which ten drops of essential oil have been added. Occasionally neat oil on a small compress can be very effective, especially for abscesses and bruises.

SURROUND YOURSELF WITH SCENT

Essential oil burners allow you to perfume a room and improve your well-being at the same time. Depending on the oil you choose you can create a warm, relaxing atmosphere or a refreshing, zesty, uplifting one. Also, by using eucalyptus oil, say, in the burner you can relieve cold symptoms and help keep the germs at bay from others in your home.

MASSAGE

This is the most relaxing, and therapeutic, way of all to experience aromatherapy. Essential oils are blended and then worked into the body using massage techniques that stimulate the whole system while improving the circulation and relaxing the nervous system. A professional aromatherapy treatment usually lasts for around one and a half hours and is a wonderful experience that I would recommend to anyone.

It's possible for you to enjoy giving and receiving massage using essential oils, and I go into more detail about this later in this book. Give it a try. You'll find even giving a simple massage can be very relaxing.

WHERE DO THESE OILS COME FROM?

By now, you may be wondering how these potent little oils are produced. As I mentioned before, they are obtained from different parts of plants, shrubs and trees and the amount of essential oil in each plant is minute. Just imagine: it takes 2,000 pounds (900 kilos) of rose petals to produce just 1 pound (½ kilo) of rose oil!

Try squeezing the peel of any citrus fruit, such as a lemon or orange, and you will extract a tiny amount of essential oil. This is called hand expression and it is still used today to extract citrus oils. The oil is collected into a sponge which is then squeezed into a container when saturated.

The most popular method of extraction nowadays is distillation. The oil-bearing parts of the chosen plant, for example the flowers and leaves, are packed into a distillating vessel which is then closed and boiled with water. The boiling water causes the oil cells to burst. The oil and water separate and the essential oil can then be drawn off. There are different methods of distillation, including steam and dry distillation.

The water separated from the oil always carries the oil's fragrance and is often sold as a separate product. You may have used rosewater or orange flower water as a skin freshener, or perhaps even as a flavouring for cakes and desserts.

If you think about it, it is easy to see why the oils vary so much in availability and price. For instance, lavender is easy to grow and has a high yield of flowers, making lavender oil reasonably priced. On the other hand, roses have a very low oil yield, making rose oil one of the most expensive to produce. In fact, both rose and jasmine oil are truly worth more than their weight in gold!

The quality of the oil is also influenced by the climatic and soil conditions in which the plant has grown. French and English lavender therefore produce slightly different oils.

HOW TO RECOGNIZE AN ESSENTIAL OIL

A selection of essential oils is now available from health food shops, chemists and by mail order. When you are buying them, be careful to choose essential oils, not perfumed oils. Although these may well smell delicious they are not beneficial for aromatherapy.

An essential oil is:
☆ Thin and watery rather than oily
☆ Swift to evaporate and it won't leave a greasemark on paper
☆ Overpoweringly scented when neat, which can be quite unpleasant

Perfumed oils will always smell pleasant whereas essential oils often have more of the effect of smelling salts.

All essential oils fall into three basic categories:

Top notes These oils evaporate very quickly. They are generally uplifting and stimulating, with a greenish, fresh aroma.

Middle notes These are used to help with most bodily functions and the body's metabolism.

Base notes These are extremely relaxing, sometimes sedative and generally have a lovely, warm aroma.

You'll notice essential oils are always sold in tinted glass bottles (if not, be suspicious). This is because they are special oils that need a little care. They are damaged by light and should always be stored in a dark, cool place. Be careful to keep the lids tightly screwed on your bottles, otherwise you will be disappointed to discover your oils have evaporated into thin air.

CARRIER OILS

Pure essential oils are hardly ever used neat but instead are blended into a carrier oil. This does just what the name suggests: it acts as a base for the essential oil and is a lubricant, so making massage easier and more effective.

Carrier oils are always vegetable in origin. They

should be natural, unprocessed oils which have not been treated with chemicals. Any vegetable oil can be used as a carrier but some are more suitable than others. For instance, virgin olive oil could be used but its smell would overpower your chosen essential oil and also it is quite expensive.

I suggest you try raiding your food cupboards! Look for an oil which is fine-textured with little or no colour or smell. I find the following are ideal as general carrier oils and are all easily available in most supermarkets and health food shops.

☆ Soya bean oil
☆ Grapeseed oil
☆ Safflower oil
☆ Sunflower oil

If your skin is very dry, richer vegetable oils can be mixed with any of the above oils. Avocado oil is very lubricating, or you could try sweet almond oil. Wheatgerm oil is excellent for helping to heal scar tissue or for very dehydrated skin. However, it tends to have a rather bready smell so be careful to mix it with one of the plainer carrier oils. Wheatgerm oil acts as a preservative, too, so add a few drops of it when mixing a blend of essential oils into a carrier oil to prolong the shelf life.

BLENDING

A general rule of thumb for blending in aromatherapy is to use six drops of an essential oil to every 2 tsp (10 ml) of carrier oil. If blending the oils to use on your face I would suggest that you decrease the amount of essential oil to four drops.

Remember, essential oils are most potent in very small quantities. Adding more than a few drops to your carrier oil will not increase their beneficial effect and could even do the exact opposite. A little essential oil will go a long, long way.

Blending is fun, and there is no end to the experimenting you can do. (An egg cup is the ideal mixing container.) Last winter I found a mixture of orange, cinnamon and clove oils gave a lovely, spicy Christmas aroma and so used it as a room scenter during the festive season. It's a good idea to label your blends once you have mixed them, as it is not easy to recognize the individual essential oils once several have been blended together. Also, you should date the bottle and try to use the contents within a couple of months while they are still fresh.

Actually, it is interesting to try to decipher the different aromas in a blend. Try it! Usually, the top note oil will be the one you pick out first as this is the most volatile. Middle notes can be harder to determine. Base notes come through last, and are heavy and warm smelling. In time you'll find it easier to pick out the individual aromas, rather like a wine taster with various wines.

When I was training I remember one of the tutors chose an oil to suit the personality of each student on her course. I found this quite fascinating, and often now find myself doing the same thing with clients. I was melissa, by the way — a very cheering oil sometimes called heart's delight or the elixir of life. It is a good general tonic that has been used medicinally for several hundred years. Once you have become familiar with the different oils, you might like to see which oil most matches your personality, and then go on to pair up oils with the characters of your family and friends. You will find it fascinating and so will they!

Chapter 2

ESSENTIAL OILS AND THEIR POWERS

A

Antiseptic All essential oils are antiseptic and are a useful addition to your first aid kit.

B

Benzoin This is actually a tree resin which is processed to turn it into a liquid. You may already be familiar with benzoin in the form of friar's balsam, but it is also used to make incense.

Helpful for:

Coughs, colds and flu Try steam inhalation.

Stiff or aching joints Mix into a carrier oil and massage into the problem area, or use on a compress.

Nervous exhaustion, tension Mix into a carrier oil and use for massage particularly around the neck and shoulder area.

Sore, dry skin Mix into a carrier oil (wheatgerm oil is good) and apply to the affected area at

	regular intervals. You can also add it to your bath.
Itchy skin, dermatitis	Mix into a carrier oil or a perfume-free cream and apply to the affected area.

| **Bergamot** | This is a member of the citrus family, and the oil is extracted by pressing the peel of the fruit. Bergamot essence is used to make Earl Grey tea and gives it its characteristic perfume. Bergamot is a powerful antiseptic and an appetite stimulant. It must not be used neat on the skin because it can cause pigmentation marks. |

Helpful for:

Cold sores	Blend into a carrier oil and apply to the cold sore with a cotton bud every few hours.
Oily, spotty skin	Blend into a carrier oil (wheatgerm oil is good) and massage into the affected area. You can also steam your face with bergamot mixed with boiling water.
Psoriasis	Blend into a carrier oil (evening primrose oil is helpful for psoriasis) and massage into the affected area, or add to the bathwater.
Cystitis	Add to the bathwater and soak in it for 15 minutes.

C

| **Camomile** | The camomile family is large and there are several different camomile essential oils. German camomile is the most |

expensive, but all camomile oils are helpful for sensitive conditions and can be used safely for children. Camomile tea is widely available, and the plant feverfew — belonging to the camomile family — is now being used to help migraine sufferers.

Helpful for:

Conjunc- **tivitis, sore** **eyes**
Add two drops to 2 tsp (10 ml) of cooled, boiled water. Soak cotton pads in the solution and place on the eyes, or use in an eyebath to wash the eyes.

Aches and **pains**
Blend with a carrier oil and massage into the affected area or add to the bathwater.

Hyper- **activity**
Particularly in children. Add a few drops to the bathwater, or use in a vaporizer.

Boils
Apply a small cotton compress which has been soaked in hot water and camomile and leave on until it cools.

Dermatitis, **eczema**
Blend with a carrier oil and massage into the affected area or blend with a perfume-free cream and apply regularly.

Minor skin **infections**
Apply on a cotton compress.

Insomnia
Try a camomile aromatherapy bath before bedtime. Drink camomile tea before going to bed. Use the oil in a vaporizer or sprinkle a few drops on your pillow.

Clary sage
The oil is produced from the flowers and leaves of the plant. It is mainly grown in Russia, and the oil varies greatly according to the conditions in which it is grown. Clary sage is used to make eau-de-Cologne and is very soothing used as an aftershave.

Helpful for:

Irregular, painful periods Mix into a carrier oil and massage into the lower back and lower abdomen for several days prior to, and during, your period.

Depression Add to your bath, or use in a burner or vaporizer.

Inflamed skin Particularly good for shaving rashes and inflamed skin.

Sore throat Mix into a carrier oil and rub into the chest and throat three or four times a day, or inhale.

E

Eucalyptus The eucalyptus tree is mainly found in Australia and Tasmania. The oil is extracted from the leaves by steam distillation. It has a smell you will recognize as it is often used in commercial rubs and inhalants for chest complaints and colds.

Helpful for:

Colds, sinus problems, sore throat Steam inhalation or use in an oil burner or vaporizer. Helps keep viruses at bay from other people in the home.

Muscular aches and pains Very helpful after sport or any strenuous exercise, either in the bath or in a carrier oil to massage affected areas.

Flu Mix into a carrier oil and massage well into the chest, shoulders and rib-cage.

F

Fennel

There are two types of fennel, sweet and bitter. Essential oil is extracted from the seeds, roots and leaves by steam distillation. Florence fennel is a popular vegetable often eaten with fish. It has a slightly aniseed flavour and looks rather like a very thick celery. Fennel essential oil has the same aniseed scent as the root.

Helpful for:

Flatulence   It is used to make gripe water.
Fluid   Add to the bathwater.
retention
Nausea   Add to a carrier oil and massage into the
and   stomach.
vomiting
Hiccoughs   Inhale neat from the bottle, or in steam.

G

Geranium

There are many varieties of geranium. Essential oil is usually extracted from the *Pelargonium* family, but wild geranium — known as Herb Robert — is also used. The oil is distilled from all parts of the plant. Geranium oil is a good balancer. It can uplift or have a relaxing effect and is particularly good for menopausal problems.

Helpful for:
Sore   Add two drops to a glass of warm water
throat   and use as a gargle.

Dry eczema and dermatitis	Mix into a carrier oil. If the problem is severe on the hands, try massaging with the blend, put on cotton gloves and wear overnight.
Meno-pausal bleeding	Mix into a carrier oil and massage into the lower abdomen and back. Or use a compress soaked in warm water with the geranium oil added.
Sluggish skin	Mix three or four drops into a carrier oil and use to massage the face and neck.
Nervous tension and anxiety	Use in an aromatherapy bath, or mix into a carrier oil and massage into neck and shoulders.

H

Hyssop	Hyssop is an ancient herb which was cultivated for its medicinal as well as romantic properties. The oil is extracted from the leaves and flowers by distillation. It is beneficial for all respiratory problems and can help relieve hayfever.

Helpful for:

Hayfever	Use on a handkerchief or in a vaporizer, or blend and use for facial massage.
Rheum-atism	Use in the bath or as a massage for the affected area.
Bruises	Use as a compress or gently rub over the bruised area.
Eczema	Use in a carrier oil at regular intervals.

J

Juniper

The juniper bush is found in Canada and Europe. The berries are well known as the flavouring for gin, but to make essential oil they are first dried, then distilled. Juniper oil has been used for hundreds of years as a household disinfectant.

Helpful for:

Cystitis

Blend into a carrier oil and rub the lower abdomen at regular intervals. Also add five or six drops to your bathwater and soak for at least fifteen minutes.

Period pain

Use as above.

Muscular/ rheumatic pain

Use for massage or in the bath.

Stress and anxiety

Use for massage, in the bath or in a vaporizer.

Acne

Mix four drops with 2 tsp (10 ml) of carrier oil and gently massage the face and neck (and shoulders if acne is present there).

Poor circulation

Juniper is a stimulating oil. Use in the bath, or in a carrier oil, daily to improve circulation.

Jasmine

The essential oil is extracted from the flowers of the jasmine bush. This oil has a beautiful, exotic aroma and is really helpful in cases of extreme nervous anxiety and stress. It is one of the most expensive oils and is often used in the manufacture of perfumes.

Helpful for:

Nervous exhaustion
Use in a carrier oil for massage or inhale.

Period pain
Use in a carrier oil and massage the lower abdomen and back at regular intervals.

Dry, sensitive, mature skin
Use in a carrier oil for massage or add a couple of drops to rosewater and use as a freshener.

L

Lavender
This is the great aromatherapy all-rounder. The essential oil is obtained from French and English lavender by distillation. Lavender oils blend well with other essential oils and can boost their properties. It is the most versatile oil for aromatherapy, so if in doubt, choose lavender.

Helpful for:

Acne and spotty skin
Blend in a carrier oil for massage, or add a few drops to distilled water to make a freshener.

Insect bites, stings
Dab on a few drops of neat oil.

Boils
Use neat on a small compress.

Burns
Use neat, being careful not to break the skin.

Sunburn
Mix a few drops into your aftersun lotion or a carrier oil.

Headache/ migraine
Inhale, or blend into a carrier oil and massage the face and scalp. Pay

particular attention to the temples and forehead.

Sore throat Use in a carrier oil to massage the chest and throat and/or inhale neat.

Muscular aches and pains Use to massage the affected area in a carrier oil, or add to the bath.

Irritability, tension and depression Use for masage, especially the shoulders and neck, add to the bath water or inhale.

Colds and flu Inhale, add to the bath, use in a vaporizer or use in a carrier oil to massage the head, neck and shoulders.

Indigestion, nausea Blend in a carrier oil and gently massage the stomach, or inhale.

Period pain Blend in a carrier oil and massage the lower abdomen and back. Also use in the bath.

Insect repellant Mix in a carrier oil and use on exposed areas as necessary. Use in a burner to keep insects at bay at night.

Lemon It takes 3,000 lemons to produce 2 pounds (1 kilo) of essential oil. It is extracted by pressing the rind of the fruit, which is mainly grown in Southern Italy. Hand-pressed oil is of a better quality than mechanically pressed oil. Hand pressing is a family affair. The women and children cut the lemons and scrape out the flesh, the men do the pressing.

Helpful for:
Chilblains Mix into a carrier oil and gently rub the affected areas three to four times a day.

	Or use in a footbath, soaking the feet for fifteen minutes.
Cold sores	Dab with a cotton bud which has been soaked in 2 tsp (10 ml) of boiled water to which 5 drops of oil have been added.
Bites and stings	Dab neat oil on to the bite or sting.
Mouth ulcers	Dab on the neat oil, or make a gargle adding five drops to a medium-size glass of water.
Verrucae/ warts	Dab with a cotton bud soaked in neat essential oil several times a day.
Catarrh/ colds	Mix in a carrier oil and massage the face and head, or inhale.

M

Marjoram	You may have come across this herb already — it is a popular aromatic flavouring. The oil is extracted from the plant by distillation. It has a powerful head-clearing aroma, and an uplifting effect on the spirit. Marjoram blends very well with lemon essential oil.

Helpful for:	
Anxiety and depression	Inhale, use in the bath or in a vaporizer.
Insomnia	Use in the bath or inhale.
Constipation	Blend into a carrier oil and massage into the abdomen to relieve spasm in the intestines.
Muscular aches and pains	Use in a carrier oil to massage the affected parts, or add to the bath.

Head cold   Inhale, or use to massage face and neck.

Myrrh   Myrrh essential oil is produced from the resin of the myrrh tree. It has been used since ancient Egyptian times for its rejuvenating qualities and is one of the oils used for embalming.

Helpful for:

Mouth ulcers, inflamed and sore gums   Add five drops to a medium-size glass of warm water and use as a gargle several times a day.

Cuts and grazes   Bathe the area in a solution of five drops to 2 tsp (10 ml) of cooled, boiled water.

Coughs   Blend into a carrier oil and massage the chest and throat, or inhale.

N

Niaouli   This oil is produced by steam distillation from the leaves of the niaouli tree, which is native to New Caledonia. It is an excellent antiseptic.

Helpful for:

Acne and problem skin   Blend in a carrier oil for massage, or add six drops to ½ pt (300 ml) of boiled water and use as a skin tonic.

Grazes   Dilute six drops in ½ pt (300 ml) of boiled water — very good for removing dirt from wounds.

Bronchitis, chesty cough   Inhale, or mix with a carrier oil and massage the chest.

Catarrh   Inhale.

O

Orange blossom

This essential oil is often called neroli. It is obtained from fresh orange flowers by steam distillation. If you have ever been lucky enough to see an orange blossom tree in bloom you will already know what delightful a scent it has. The tree originated in China, but is now also found in France, California and Italy. This oil is one of the most expensive, along with rose and jasmine.

Helpful for:

Sensitive skin, high colour

Blend in a carrier oil and use to massage the affected area. Or, add a few drops to a bottle of orange flower water and use as a skin tonic.

Diarrhoea

Blend in a carrier oil and massage gently into the abdomen to relieve spasms.

Shock, fear

Inhale neat oil.

Depression

Neroli is a cheering oil. Try inhaling, or add a few drops to your bathwater.

P

Petigrain

Made from the leaves of the orange blossom tree, this oil has similar properties to neroli and a pleasant, light scent. It is cheaper to produce than neroli, and often used in its place for economic reasons.

Helpful for:

Memory

Inhale neat oil.

Stress

Use in a carrier oil for massage, or in the bath.

Spotty or irritated skin   Mix with a carrier oil and use on the affected areas.

Fluid retention   Add to the bath, or mix with a carrier oil for massage.

Peppermint   The oil is obtained from the leaves and flowers by steam distillation and varies in quality depending on climatic and soil conditions. It is a very therapeutic oil which has a cooling effect on the skin and lessens pain. You'll notice most commerical indigestion cures are mint-flavoured. Peppermint is excellent for digestive problems. It also makes a great foot bath for hot, aching feet.
Note: It is not advisable to use this oil during pregnancy.

Helpful for:

Migraine   Use it neat on the temples.

Heartburn and indigestion   Mix into a carrier oil and massage the stomach and rib-cage.

Hot, aching feet   Add ten drops to a large bowl of lukewarm water. Soak feet for at least fifteen minutes.

Travel sickness   Inhale, or blend in a carrier oil and massage the stomach and temples.

Sinus, catarrh   Inhale, or use to massage the face.

Bad breath   Add five drops to ½ pt (300 ml) of water and use as a mouthwash.

R

Rosemary

A well known herb, rosemary is cultivated in France and Spain. The essential oils are distilled from the flowers and leaves. It is known as the herb for remembrance and clears the mind and stimulates the memory. It is an excellent hair tonic, improving circulation to the scalp, and is helpful for dandruff.

Helpful for:

Fainting
Inhale neat, like smelling salts.

Mental fatigue, poor memory
Inhale neat.

Dandruff, hair in poor condition
Use in a carrier oil for scalp massage. Leave for thirty minutes before shampooing.

Circulation
Use in the bath, or in a carrier oil. Rosemary has a warming, comforting effect.

Stomach pain, wind
Mix in a carrier oil and gently massage the affected area.

Rose

As I have already mentioned, this is one of the most expensive essential oils and is most used for its beautiful fragrance. It is an excellent anti-depressant, and very calming on the nervous system. I've yet to come across anyone who dislikes the aroma and effect of rose oil. Because of its cost, I wouldn't recommend the use of this oil in the bath. There are other oils you can substitute for it.

Helpful for:

Depression	Inhale, or use in a carrier oil to massage the chest, neck and face.
Irregular periods	Mix in a carrier oil and massage the abdomen and lower back daily.
Very dehydrated, mature skin	Blend with sweet almond oil and massage the face and neck, or add a few drops to your night cream. Use rosewater as a skin freshener.
Insomnia	Put a few drops on your pillow, or dab a little under your nose before retiring. **Note:** This oil can safely be used on children.

S

Sandalwood   This oil is distilled from the sandalwood tree, and the best comes from India. The wood is carved and used as a decoration in temples because of its lovely fragrance. It takes years for the trees to mature, and they are not felled until they show signs of dying. Sandalwood is a parasitic tree: it buries its roots in the roots of other trees. Sandalwood is often an ingredient of incense.

Helpful for:

Nausea, vomiting	Mix in a carrier oil and gently massage the stomach, or inhale.
Stress, tension	Inhale, use in the bath or in a burner. Can aid sleep.
Dry cough	Inhale, mix in a carrier oil and massage into the chest and throat.

Itchy, dry skin Add to your bath, or use mixed in a carrier oil. (Avocado or wheatgerm oils are very nourishing.)

Sage I'm sure you've already come across this herb as it is often used in stuffings and savoury dishes. The oil is made from the sun-dried leaves by distillation. Sage is to be found in the North Mediterranean, where it grows wild, but it is also grown as a garden herb all over the world. The essential oil is toxic in high doses, so use with care.

Helpful for:

Aching joints, rheumatism Add to your bath, or use in a carrier oil to massage the affected areas.

Nervous exhaustion A good tonic. Add to your bath, and soak for at least fifteen minutes.

Fluid retention Add to your bath, or use in a carrier oil.

Excess perspiration Dilute five drops in a glass of water. Soak cotton wool in the solution and use it under the arms and on the feet several times daily.

Sore, bleeding gums Dilute five drops in a glass of water and use as a mouthwash.

T

Tea tree The tea tree is native to Australia and the oil is distilled from the leaves. This oil is an excellent antiseptic, 12 to 15 times more potent than carbolic. When applied neat to a cut, its antiseptic potency doubles! Keep this one in your first aid box.

Helpful for:

Athlete's foot
Add six drops to a large bowl of warm water and soak feet for fifteen minutes. Repeat daily.

Boils, spots
Apply neat to the boil or spot using a cotton bud.

Thrush
Add six drops to your bath. Also, blend in a carrier oil and massage the abdomen regularly.

Cuts
Bathe with neat oil.

Sore throat
Dilute five drops in a glass of water and gargle three times a day.

Thyme
This plant has been grown for its therapeutic qualities for centuries. The essential oil is obtained from the flowering tops by steam distillation. Thyme oil stimulates white blood cell production, having an almost antibiotic effect on infections.

Helpful for:

Colds and flu
Inhale or blend with a carrier oil and use to massage the chest, neck and head. This oil can help protect others in the family from the virus. Use in a vaporizer or burner.

Sore throat, tonsillitis
Use in a gargle, two drops in a glass of water, or mix in a carrier oil and apply to the chest and throat.

Muscle fatigue
Add six drops to your bath.

Arthritis
Add to your bath, or use in a carrier oil

to rub the affected area, or make up a hot compress.

Whooping cough   Inhale, or mix into a carrier oil and rub the chest regularly.

V

Vetivert   Vetivert is a grass which grows in Indonesia and the Philippines. The oil is obtained from the root by distillation. It is popular in the perfume industry and has a long-lasting woody fragrance, often popular with men. In the East it is known as the oil of tranquility and is often used for meditation.

Helpful for:
Stress   Use in a burner or in the bath.
Tired, aching legs   Use in a carrier oil for massage.

Hysteria   Blend in a carrier oil and massage the solar plexus (see massage chapter) or inhale.
Stiff neck   Use in a carrier oil and massage the shoulders and neck.

Verbena   This oil is probably better known as lemon grass. It is a fragrant grass which grows in India, and the oil is obtained by distillation. Lemon grass is used extensively in Indian and Asian cookery and has a light, lemony scent.

Helpful for:
Acne, spotty skin   Use in a carrier oil (wheatgerm is good for its healing properties) to massage, or

dilute five drops in water and use to wipe the skin after cleansing.

Poor muscle tone Improves elasticity. Use in a carrier oil for massage, or in the bath.

Shock Inhale.

Irritability, tension Add to your bath, inhale or use in a carrier oil on the shoulders and neck.

Digestive problems e.g. colitis Use in a carrier oil to massage the abdomen at regular intervals.

Y

Ylang-ylang This tree is native to the Philippines and other parts of the Far East. The essential oil is obtained from the flowers by steam distillation. This is another oil used by the perfume industry as it has a lovely, exotic floral fragrance. It has a relaxing, sedative effect and is a pleasant oil to use in a burner to scent your home. Ylang-ylang is said to have aphrodisiac powers!

Helpful for:

Depression and nervous tension Use in a burner, the bath or for massage.

Insomnia Put a few drops on your pillow, use in the bath or a burner.

Panic, fear Inhale neat oil.

High blood pressure The oil is calming and can help to relieve high blood pressure. Use regularly in a carrier oil for massage or in the bath.

Spotty skin Use in a carrier oil, or dilute in water and use as a skin tonic.

Chapter 3

MASSAGE FOR EVERYONE

Remember how as a child if you bumped your head (or anywhere else) a wise adult would kindly rub it better? Or that if any part of your body aches now it's instinctive to put your hand there?

Very simply, this is how massage works. Touch is both healing and comforting and, what's more, we can all enjoy the pleasures of it — both giving and receiving. Massage is beneficial to us in several different ways and:

☆ Improves blood circulation
☆ Calms the nervous system
☆ Stimulates skin function
☆ Improves muscle tone
☆ Eases aches and pains in muscles and joints

And it feels marvellous!

THE BASIC PRINCIPLES OF MASSAGE

In basic terms massage is a way of stroking the body, with variations in the length and depth of strokes. However, you should always direct firm strokes towards the heart, as this will be beneficial to the circulation.

Long flowing massage strokes with little pressure on the body are the most soothing and relaxing. This type of movement is called *effleurage*. It is done with the whole hand using gentle, even pressure and is often used to start and finish a massage.

Patting or tapping the skin with your fingers quickly and slowly is stimulating and helps to increase blood flow. This is called *tapotement*. It is usually done on small areas such as the forehead, cheeks and neck.

Petrissage involves squeezing and releasing a muscle or part of a muscle group. A good example of this kind of movement is kneading dough. It is mostly done with both hands, particularly on the thighs and buttocks. Petrissage helps strengthen muscle fibre, remove waste products and ease fatigue.

There's another type of massage movement called *friction* which creates just that. It involves rubbing the hands backwards and forwards across an area and is very warming and stimulating to the tissues. Rubbing our hands quickly together on a freezing winter day is a good example of how friction can work.

A professional aromatherapist uses mainly effleurage and works on pressure points with some frictions and petrissage, but there is no reason why you can't vary the movements if you decide you would like to try giving a simple massage.

You don't need to be an expert to give a soothing massage to family or friends. Once you've learned a few basic movements you'll probably be in demand.

DOS AND DON'TS

Massage is a gentle healing art suitable for everyone from babies to the very elderly. However, there are certain times or conditions when it should be avoided (for example, when the person has just eaten a heavy meal). Often, this just means leaving out a body area but use your common sense and if unsure leave well alone.

Do not massage:
☆ Any infected area
☆ A person who is feverish or has a raised temperature
☆ Over an area where varicose veins are present
☆ Over any unusual swelling or inflammation
☆ Bruised or broken skin

Before massaging do:
☆ Check with the person about to be massaged whether any of the above apply
☆ Make sure the room is warm enough
☆ Warm your hands before massaging — cold hands are a real shock. Not a good way to begin!

CREATING THE RIGHT ATMOSPHERE

Wouldn't it be wonderful to be massaged in a tropical country, with the warm sun beating down, soft sounds of the sea in the background and the sweet scents of flowers occasionally wafting over you?

Well, perhaps it's rather a far-fetched dream but it is still possible to create a lovely, relaxing atmosphere at home, especially with the help of aromatherapy oils. I think the most important consideration is that the room, or area, you use to give a massage is really warm. Believe me, there's nothing more miserable than receiving a soothing massage while shivering and covered with goose pimples. Remember that while a person is lying still he or she generates less body heat: you know how difficult it is to get off to sleep if you feel really cold in bed.

It's a good idea to have a blanket, or large towel, so you can cover the parts of the body you are not working on. Also, it feels good to be wrapped up while being massaged. If you like, you can even wrap a hot water bottle in a towel and pop it under your patient's feet for a really luxurious treat.

Harsh, bright lights are unpleasant when being massaged. Obviously, until you feel confident in what you are doing you'll need a reasonable amount of light, just to see clearly as you go. A table lamp is sufficient for this: it gives a softer, gentler light than overhead lighting. Once you feel happy about your massage movements you can work by candlelight. The soft flickering of the flames has a soothing, hypnotic effect which is really relaxing.

Try to keep noise to the minimum, and close the curtains or blinds. This helps to cut out traffic noise. If you think you may be disturbed, unplug the telephone. It's now possible to buy some really interesting tapes to play in the background. Sounds of the sea, tinkling bells, birdsong and running water all combined with gentle, lulling music can take you off into a dreamlike state.

Part of the benefits of aromatherapy massage is the feeling of getting away from stressful day-to-day living, so music can be a great help in creating a relaxing atmosphere. This is a very personal thing and you'll find out for yourself which sounds are most relaxing for you. I find playing the tapes helps me to relax more while I am giving a massage, too, even when the day has been hectic and I am feeling less than calm.

Aromatherapy oils are marvellous for creating different atmospheres in the home and are much more authentic than using chemical copies or perfume sprays. Smells seem to strongly imprint themselves on our memories, and a certain aroma can evoke all sorts of feelings from the past. For example, the smell of warm spices, such as cinnamon and cloves, always reminds me of Christmasses spent at my grandparents'. And the sweet, sickly scent of benzoin reminds me of the day my little sister drank half a bottle of friar's balsam thinking it was some sort of chocolate drink!

There are several ways of scenting your home with essential oils. The simplest is probably to add a few drops of your chosen oil to a small bowl of water and then stand it over a radiator. The essential oil floats on the water and gradually evaporates into the air, aided by the heat.

A more sophisticated method is to use an oil burner or vaporizer. These come in many different designs, but with the oil burners there is no need to use any water. You just put a few drops of essential oil into the top of the burner, then light a night light underneath. Vaporizers usually have a deeper dish into which you add water, followed by your favourite essential oil. However, whether you use an oil burner or a vaporizer, do be careful not to let it burn dry!

Used in this way the oils can become mood enhancers. They can remove stale smells or even help with conditions such as headaches, colds or insomnia.

Another way to perfume a room is to make your own pot-pourri. Gather flowers and herbs from your garden and hang them up in bundles to dry. (The airing cupboard is the ideal place for this.) Once dried, crumble them together, keeping some of the smaller flower heads intact. Now you are ready to perfume your pot-pourri with the essential oils of your choice. Generally, I find it better to use single essences rather than a blend.

Here are a few suggestions:
Fresh and light Lemon, coriander, vetivert and melissa
Warm and spicy Benzoin, cinnamon, clove and patchouli
Sweet and flowery Lavender, neroli, ylang-ylang, sandalwood

You can also boost a tired pot-pourri by using aromatherapy oils in the same way.

Another way to perfume a room is with a light bulb

ring. This is either a ceramic or metal ring which sits on a light bulb. Once the ring is in place all you do is pour in a few drops of essential oil. The fragrance is more effective when the light is turned on as the heat increases the oil's evaporation.

Now you have a few ideas on how to create a warm, relaxing atmosphere for aromatherapy massage we can look at the massage techniques in more detail. As I mentioned before, everyone can learn to give a simple massage; you'll be surprised at how enjoyable it can be.

SIMPLE BODY MASSAGE STEP-BY-STEP

Just before you begin your massage check that your hands are clean and your nails fairly short with no jagged edges. Take off any rings if you wear them. You will find if you use aromatherapy oils regularly that your nails strengthen and your hands become smoother and more supple. Also, check with your massage partner to make sure there are no reasons to stop you going ahead.

THE FEET

Probably the most neglected part of our bodies, feet deserve a loving massage from time to time. Make sure your partner is warm and comfortable. Uncover one foot by folding back the towel or blanket. Now pour a little of your chosen oil into the palm of one hand. Rub your hands together to evenly distribute the oil. Now you are ready to begin.

1. Enclose the foot between both hands (one on top, one underneath), then gently slide your hands off the foot coming forward to the toes. This movement should be slow and soothing. Repeat four or five times.

2. Gently circle around the ankles using your thumbs. This area can be tender, so go easy.

3. Rub over the top of the foot with your thumbs in little circles, coming down from the ankle area to the toes. Repeat three or four times.

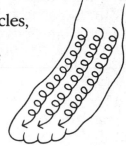

4. Now rub each toe with the same little circular movements.

5. Rotate each toe twice in each direction.

6. Gently pull each toe between finger and thumb.

7. Zigzag down the sole of the foot from toes to heel with your thumbs overlapped.

8. Enclose the foot in your hands then rub them in opposite directions, to create frictions. This is very warming.

9. Hold the foot firmly and slowly rotate the ankle clockwise then anti-clockwise. Repeat a couple of times.

10. Repeat step 1.

Once completed, wrap the foot up again for warmth and repeat the movements on the other foot. By now your massage partner will be feeling more relaxed and at ease with your touch.

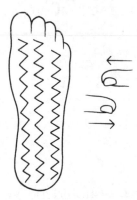

THE LOWER LEGS AND KNEES

Warm a little oil in your hands.

1. With one hand behind the other, smooth the oil on to the front of the leg, starting at the top of the foot and working up to the knee. This movement distributes the oil and soothes and relaxes the whole area.
2. Rub across the front of the leg using both hands to create frictions. This increases the blood circulation to the area and reduces aches and pains.
3. Lift the leg up so the knee is bent. Squeeze and relax rhythmically down the muscles of the calf from knee to ankle. Repeat several times. Put the leg down.
4. Work around the kneecap in little circular motions with both hands. Be careful not to use too much pressure.
5. Now using your thumbs gently slide them around each side of the kneecap.
6. Stretch out your thumbs from your fingers to create an arch. Sweep over the whole knee using alternate hands several times.

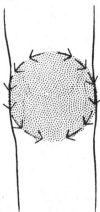

Now wrap up the lower leg and proceed to the thigh.

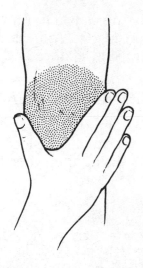

THE UPPER LEGS

1. Apply oil as for the lower leg.
2. Glide up the leg from knee to groin, using one hand behind the other. This movement should be fairly slow and rhythmical. Make sure your movements cover the whole of the thigh area. Repeat four to five times.
3. Stroke the upper inner thigh diagonally from knee to groin hand over hand. Repeat four or five times.
4. Squeeze and release rhythmically first along the inner thigh from knee to groin, then along the outer thigh.
5. Using your knuckles rake quickly up from the knee to the groin, taking in the whole thigh area. This is a friction movement and increases the surface blood circulation. You'll notice the skin colours quite quickly and feels warmer to the touch.
6. Uncover the lower leg, then effleurage the whole leg from foot to groin as in step 2.
7. Finish off by enclosing the foot in your hands a couple of times. Cover the leg then repeat all the movements on the other one.

By now you'll find your hands have become more sensitive to your partner and you'll notice differences in the skin texture and muscle tone.

THE HANDS AND ARMS

1. Smooth on the oil as before. When working on the arm it's easier to effleurage with one hand only, using the other to hold the arm steady.

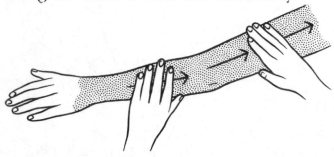

2. Bend the arm at the elbow. Massage around the wrist with little thumb circles using both hands.
3. Work down from the wrist to the ends of the fingers using little thumb circles. Repeat five times.
4. Stretch each finger, then thumb, in turn between your finger and thumb.
5. Rotate the fingers and thumb first clockwise then anti-clockwise.

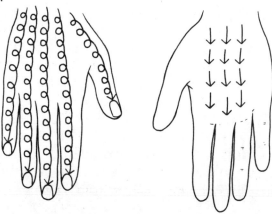

6. Turn the hand over and rub gently along the solar plexus (from centre wrist down the palm to the middle finger) using alternate thumbs. This is calming to the nervous system.
7. Rotate the hand at the wrist clockwise then anti-clockwise. To do this lock your fingers into your partner's.
8. Turn the hand over and work on the inside of the wrist up to the elbow using alternate sweeping movements. Repeat four or five times.
9. Bend the arm at the elbow and bring the lower arm up and across the chest. Squeeze all along the upper arm from elbow to shoulder using both hands.
10. Bring the arm back down to the side then effleurage the whole area from hand to shoulder four or five times. Cover the arm and repeat on the other side.

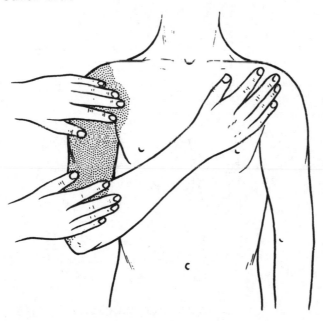

THE ABDOMEN

The abdomen is a soft area protecting vital organs, so please be gentle. Fold the towel or blanket down to expose the area from just below the breasts to a couple of inches (centimetres) below the navel.

1. Apply oil, starting just under the rib-cage, working down and out towards the waist. Be careful to keep your hands relaxed and contoured to your partner. Poking fingers feel very uncomfortable here.
2. With one hand on top of the other 'iron' around the lower abdomen in large circles. Keep the pressure light and even.
3. Fan your hands out and work from the navel out to the waist. Slide your hands under the waist then gently pull them back round to the front again. Repeat several times.

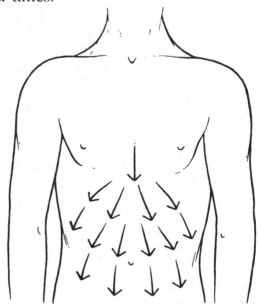

4. Stroke diagonally with alternate hands from the waist down to below the navel, first on the left side, then on the right.

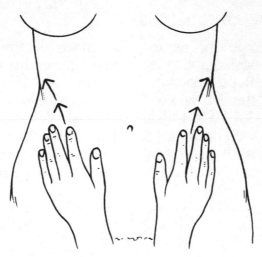

5. Stroke down from the solar plexus to the navel, one hand behind the other, to finish off this area.

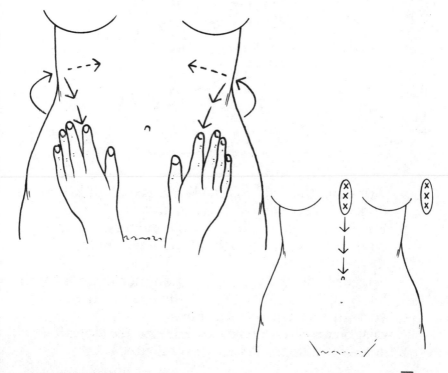

THE BACKS OF THE LEGS

1. Effleurage oil as for the front of the legs but working from the foot right up to the top of the thigh. Repeat four or five times.
2. Bend the leg at the knee, supporting it with one hand. Stroke firmly down the calf, across behind the knee, then back up to the foot several times keeping your hands contoured to the leg. Put the leg down.

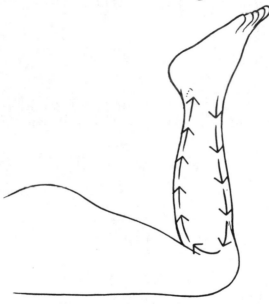

3. Work up the calf to the knee, using little circles. Repeat several times to cover the whole calf.
4. Using your index and middle fingers, make small circular movements behind the knee. Be careful not to press too hard.
5. Squeeze rhythmically along the inner thigh from the knee upwards. Repeat on the outer thigh, doing each movement several times.
6. Diagonally stroke from the inner knee upwards and across the thigh. Repeat several times.

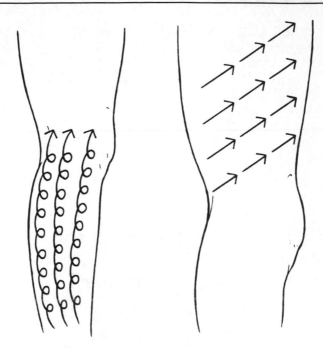

7. Finish by effleuraging the whole leg several times, from foot to thigh. Wrap up and repeat on the other leg.

THE BACK

Don't be at all surprised if your massage partner dozes off at this point. Back massage is extremely soothing and relaxing and great for relieving stress and tension.

Uncover the back to just show the buttock crease. At this point it is a good idea to place a small rolled-up towel under your partner's forehead otherwise he or she will have to turn his or her head sideways or end up with a squashed nose through which it is difficult to breathe.

1. Starting at the lower back effleurage oil using both hands. Work slowly up the back to the shoulders,

pressing gently on the upward strokes, releasing the pressure as you come back down.

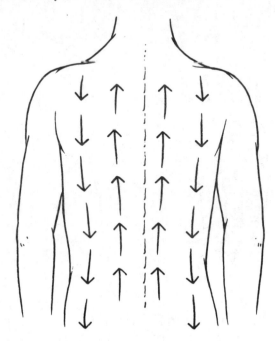

2. Starting at the base of the spine work up on either side, using gentle thumb pressure or little thumb circles. Repeat five or six times.

3. With reinforced hands (one on top of the other) sweep up the spine then work around the shoulder blades in a figure-of-eight movement. Repeat the figure-of-eight four or five times.

4. Now work around each shoulder blade individually, still with reinforced hands, in a circular motion. Repeat four or five times each side. You may feel knots (little bumps) around the shoulder blades. These are an indication of tension, and massage here gives great relief.

5. Work around the shoulder blades with your thumbs,

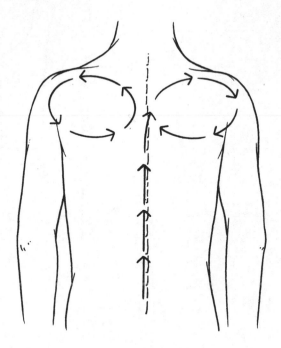

helping to break down the knots and bumps. Allow your partner to be your guide as these areas can be tender.

6. Squeeze along the top of the shoulders from the neck out, using your fingers and thumbs. Repeat four to five times on each side.
7. Stroke up the back of the neck and out to the ears, using your thumbs.
8. Stand at your partner's head and sweep your hands down the centre back, across the top of the buttocks, then firmly pull up at the sides. Repeat five times.
9. Move to your partner's side and rub backwards and forwards over the whole back with frictions to warm the area.
10. Make thumb circles out from just above the buttock crease round towards the hips. This area can often

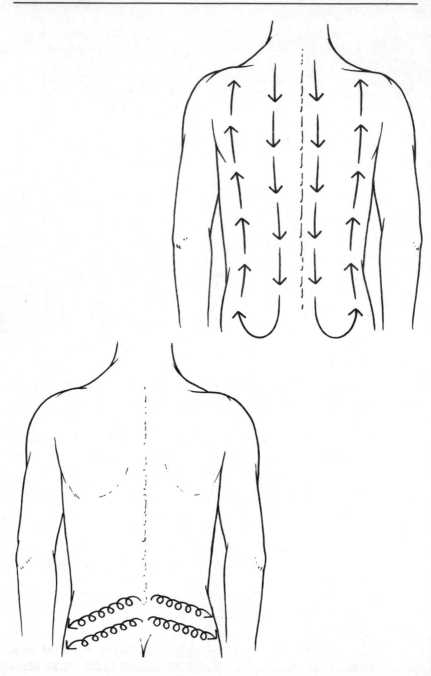

be tender and massage here is soothing. Repeat several times.

11. Effleurage the whole back.
12. Gently stroke up the spine, hand over hand, several times, allowing your touch to get lighter and lighter.
13. Finish by gently holding your partner. Place one hand at the base of the spine, the other at the base of the neck. Hold this position and feel the warmth build up under your hands. After approximately one minute gently lift your hands off. Cover your partner over.

By now, he or she might be snoozing!

THE SHOULDERS AND NECK

If your partner is feeling very tense, and you haven't time to give a full body massage, working on the shoulders and neck will still offer great relief. For this your partner should be lying on his or her back. Uncover the chest by folding down the towel or blanket.

1. Apply oil to your partner's chest, shoulders and neck.
2. Begin effleuraging by placing both hands on the upper chest, fingers facing towards each other. Now, slowly pull your hands across the chest and out to the shoulders. Curve your hands round the shoulders and under them, then bring your hands in to meet at the back of the neck. Stroke up the neck to the base of the skull. Repeat four or five times.
3. Gently knuckle the chest and shoulders in the sequence shown in the diagram on the left. To knuckle make your hands into relaxed fists, and move the knuckles in circular movements. This sounds more difficult than it is.
4. Gently turn your partner's head to one side. Stroke along the top of the shoulder and the side of the

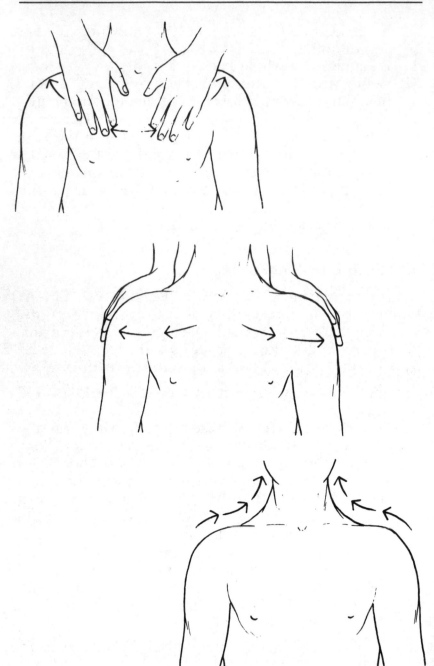

neck with your first three fingers. Repeat three times.

5. Repeat the above sequence, but circle your fingers this time. Do this three times.

6. Turn your partner's head to the other side and repeat movements 4 and 5. Return the head to the centre.

7. Slide your hands down your partner's back as far as you can comfortably reach. Find the groove each side of the spine with your fingers. Pull your hands up the spine with a little pressure on the groove each side. Repeat three times.

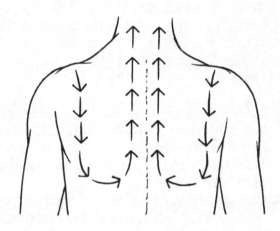

8. Now you are going to stretch the neck — these movements stretch out the muscles of the shoulders and neck and ease tension. If your partner is relaxed you'll find you will take all the weight of the head. If he or she is tense, go easy and make the movements slow and gentle. You don't want any pulled muscles.

9. Cup both hands under your partner's head, your fingers resting in the base of the skull. Lift the head slightly, then gently pull towards you. Lower the head slowly, then repeat.

10. Hold the back of the head in one hand and move it slowly towards the left shoulder while gently pressing down on the right shoulder with your other hand. Bring the head back to the centre and then repeat on the other side.
11. Finish with some effleurage movements as you began.

THE FACE AND SCALP

Until you've had the pleasurable experience of a face massage you probably won't have realized how much tension we hold in our faces. Think of frowning — this is caused by muscle action, and these muscles tire just as much as those of any other part of the body. A caring face massage can smooth away some of this tension, leaving us looking (and feeling) more at ease and relaxed.

Offer to take your partner's hair off the face with a headband, as it will inevitably get a little oily around the hairline during the massage. Be careful not to use too much oil on the face or you'll find it difficult to massage specific areas without slipping.

Encourage your partner to close his or her eyes, so as to focus on your touch. Also, it can be disconcerting to have someone staring up at you, especially as a novice.

1. Begin by stroking up each side of the jawline to the forehead. Repeat four or five times.
2. Slowly stroke the forehead rhythmically with the flat of your hand from just above the brows to the hairline.
3. Starting at the centre hairline slide your thumbs out to the side, applying gentle pressure. Move down the forehead slightly and repeat. Continue this outward stroking pressure until you reach the eyebrows.

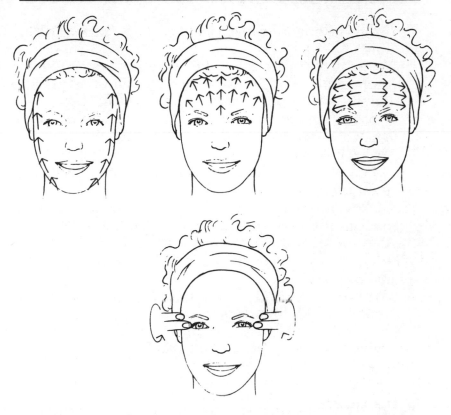

4. Now place the heel of each hand on the centre forehead and slide out to the sides. Repeat three times.
5. Place the first two fingers of each hand on the temples and circle gently for a minute or two, applying a little pressure.

All the above movements help to relieve a headache. Try lavender oil for your massage, as I've found it can ward off a headache if used in time.

6. Place your thumbs on your partner's inner eyebrows and slide out to the sides. Repeat three times.
7. With your index finger and thumb gently pull along the brow bone. Repeat three times.
8. Stroke gently over the eyelids with your ring fingers,

from the inner to the outer corners. Repeat three times.

9. Alternately stroke down the nose with your thumbs, then gently rub round the nose tip and nostrils. Be careful not to press hard on the nostrils.
10. Stroke the cheeks across the cheekbones and gradually work down the face to the chin.
11. Make little circular movements across the top lip. When you reach the corner of the mouth lift slightly, then repeat.
12. Make pinching movements out along the jawline and up towards the ears.
13. Rub the earlobes between your fingers and thumb, then gently pinch all around the outer ear. Most people love this.
14. Sweep your hands up the neck and on to the cheeks. Hold, then repeat.
15. Finish by stroking the forehead, getting lighter and lighter until you bring your hands off.

SCALP MOVEMENTS

1. Remove your partner's headband. Bring your hands up the side of the face to the forehead, then rake them through the hair. Repeat several times.
2. 'Glue' your fingers onto the scalp and move it around against the skull. Move your fingers to a different position and repeat this process until all the scalp has been covered.
3. Rub vigorously over the scalp, as if shampooing the hair.
4. Take little bunches of hair all over the scalp and tug gently. This feels lovely and really stimulates the scalp.
5. Repeat step 1 to finish off.

SELF-MASSAGE

Although not as relaxing as receiving a massage, self-massage is a helpful technique and can be practised whenever you feel achy, tired or stiff. By trying self-massage you will more fully appreciate the way your touch can be healing. After all, you will know exactly where the pain is, or how deep to work on a particularly stiff area.

THE FEET

Work on the feet as described in the step-by-step massage. It's easiest to work sitting on the floor with your legs outstretched.

THE LEGS

Sit on the floor with your legs outstretched. Bend your right leg at the knee.
1. Effleurage the front, then back, of your lower leg several times.
2. Friction rub briskly up and down all over the front and back of the lower leg. You'll soon feel the warmth this produces as it really whips up your circulation.

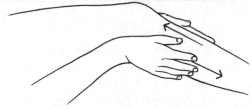

3. Work on the knee as in the step-by-step massage.
4. Lower your leg, then effleurage the thigh.
5. Quickly rake up the thigh with your fingertips, using both hands. This increases the circulation.

6. Squeeze and release along the inner thigh, then the outer thigh.
7. Do diagonal stroking as in the step-by-step massage.
8. Finish with effleurage. Repeat on the other leg.

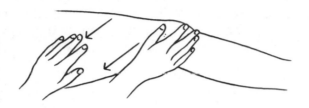

THE TUMMY

1. Stroke down from the solar plexus hand behind hand to your navel.
2. Stroke down from the solar plexus, tracing your rib-cage to your waistline with both hands.
3. With hands reinforced 'iron' in circles all over the abdomen with even pressure.
4. Squeeze up each side from your hipbones past your waist.
5. Rub backwards and forwards across your lower abdomen.
6. Repeat step 1.

THE HIPS AND BUTTOCKS

Lie on one side with your knees bent.
1. Stroke round from your hipbone to your coccyx (sitting bone), then down and round the buttock before finishing at the hip.
2. Squeeze and release on the buttock to improve circulation and tone muscle.
3. Gently pinch all over buttocks.
4. Finish by stroking the whole area.

THE ARMS AND HANDS

Follow the sequence in the step-by-step massage. This is easiest lying down.

THE CHEST

1. Still lying down, massage up from between your ribs across to your shoulders.
2. Gently press along your collarbone with your fingertips.
3. Stroke down between your breasts and out to the sides across the rib-cage.

THE SHOULDERS AND NECK

1. Lying down, massage across your upper chest and across and round your shoulders.
2. Turn your head to one side and work up your neck with your hand cupped. Repeat several times on both sides.
3. Work up between your shoulder blades to the base of your skull. Repeat several times.

THE BACK

You'll need to sit upright for this one!
1. Reach around with both hands, and starting below the waist work up as far as you can.
2. Try thumb pressures on your spine, if you can reach, having your fingers pointing forwards. Pressing the lower back and sacrum (top of buttocks) area really relieves backache.
3. Alternatively, try using a wooden back massage roller or wriggle around with your back against a rolling pin.

THE FACE AND SCALP

Face

1. Stroke all over your face and forehead.
2. Massage your temples with the fingertips of both hands.
3. Gently smooth over your eyelids from the inner to outer corners with your thumbs.
4. Press with your thumbs just below the inner eyebrow corner. Release, then repeat. Do this three or four times.
5. Stroke down the sides of your face to the jawline.
6. Pinch all along your jawline from ear to ear.
7. Finish face by repeating step 1.

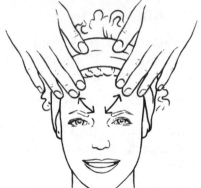

Scalp

1. Massage your scalp as if shampooing your hair.
2. Lock your fingers on to your scalp and move it over your skull. These movements increase the blood circulation and, done regularly, will improve the condition of your hair.
3. Gently tug sections of your hair all over your head. Finish your self-massage by lying down and completely relaxing, hands open at your sides, and breathing deeply for a minute or two. Depending on which oil you have chosen, you'll feel deeply relaxed, maybe a little sleepy or invigorated and energized.

Chapter 4

AROMABEAUTY

Beauty is really, I believe, the art of making the most of ourselves. Our skin and hair reflect the way we are — either glowing and vital when we are physically well and fairly at peace with the world, or dull and grey, and rather drawn, when we have been ill, are feeling off par, or suffering from the effects of stress or worry.

A healthy, balanced diet, exercise, relaxation and sufficient sleep are just as important as a sensible skin and hair care routine. Remember! Beauty begins on the inside.

As I've already shown you earlier in this book, aromatherapy can help you to alleviate the problems associated with stress, fatigue and some illnesses. Aromatherapy can also help you to care for your skin, and in a positive way can improve your beauty routine.

Aromatherapy allows you to tailor your skin, hair and body care to your individual requirements. It's a simple way of introducing effective treatments for your face and body without having to buy lots and lots of different products: you can adapt the ones you already have with aromatherapy oils.

Mixing aromatherapy oils into your own creams and lotions is rewarding and enjoyable. You'll soon realize how much you can improve your overall appearance and well-being without too much fuss and expense. Also, you'll benefit from the soothing aromas of the oils.

DO YOU KNOW YOUR SKIN TYPE?

Oily skin

☆ Feels supple and elastic, even after washing
☆ Looks shiny
☆ Often blackheads and/or spots present
☆ Can look sluggish, sallow
☆ Hair is often oily, too

Oily skin, when properly looked after, can be an advantage. It stays elastic and firm for longer and is less prone to wrinkles and fine lines than other skin types. However, it needs special attention to keep it free from spots and blackheads, and can sometimes look rather dull and yellow.

Dry skin

☆ Feels tight after washing
☆ Is dry, scaly or flaky to the touch
☆ Can look grey or pinkish
☆ Reacts adversely to harsh products

Dry skin is clear of spots and in younger years is fairly problem-free. Because it is not well lubricated naturally, it ages more quickly, so extra care must be taken with moisturizers. It's a good idea to use a sunscreen all year round to reduce the harsh, drying effects of ultra violet rays.

Hyper-sensitive skin

☆ Usually fair, freckly or prone to high colour
☆ Burns easily in sunlight
☆ Flushes quickly

☆ Reacts to harsh substances quickly, becoming itchy, red and irritated

This skin type is often found in blondes and redheads. Extra care must be taken when choosing skin care products so they protect and soothe, rather than irritate, this type of skin.

Combination skin

☆ Spots/blemishes on nose, chin or forehead
☆ Blackheads on nose, chin or forehead
☆ Dry patches, particularly cheeks
☆ Cheeks feel tight after washing
☆ Shiny patches and flaky patches

Combination skin is the most common. It's important to treat the oily and dry areas differently, as a product for oily skin can be damaging to the dryer, sensitive areas.

Normal skin

☆ Clear and free of spots and blemishes
☆ Soft and supple
☆ Even texture and colour

This is very rare, if not non-existent, except on babies and young children and a few fortunate adults. If you are lucky enough to have inherited this skin type, remember it still needs to be looked after.

Still not sure which of the above applies to you? Try this simple test:

1. On waking (presuming you cleansed your face the night before and didn't use a greasy night cream), take a paper tissue and separate its layers so you have just one ply.

2. Press this on to your face, touching all the contours.
3. Hold it up to the light. Any oily areas will show up on the tissue.

Results

No oil marks — dry skin, maybe sensitive, too.
Oil marks down centre of tissue — combination skin.
Mainly oily — oily skin.

CLEANSE, BALANCE, MOISTURIZE

Once you have decided on your skin type, you can begin an effective routine to keep your skin feeling healthy and looking great.

Cleansing

I'd like to point out that an effective cleansing routine will balance your skin, helping it to function properly. You don't want to make it squeaky clean. This kind of over-cleansing takes away the skin's natural protective barrier (called the acid mantle) and leaves it more susceptible to the effects of bacteria and environmental influences such as dust and pollution.

All skin types need to be cleansed twice a day. As a beauty therapist I've found a lot of clients who wouldn't dream of going to bed without cleansing their skins, but don't bother in the mornings. However, cleansing in the morning is really important. Your skin throws out toxic waste products while you sleep, and if you apply moisturizer straight on to your skin you are actually preventing this shedding process from being effective.

Oily skin cleansing

Morning Either use a cleansing milk or a balanced cleansing bar, if you prefer to wash your face.

Evening First, use a cleansing milk to remove all traces of make-up. Then, wash your face with a balanced cleansing bar.

Note: Just washing your face is not an effective way of removing make-up.

Combination skin cleansing

Morning As for oily skin, paying particular attention to nose, chin and forehead areas.

Evening As for oily skin, but be gentle on your cheeks and if they are dry repeat the cleansing process with a milk cleanser rather than by washing your face.

Dry skin cleansing

Morning Use a cleansing cream. Massage it into your face with your fingers thoroughly, then remove.

Evening Use cleansing milk to remove make-up. Cleanse again using cleansing cream.

Hyper-sensitive skin cleansing

Morning Use a cleansing milk or cream specially made for very sensitive skin. Avoid skin washes.

Evening Remove make-up with a cleansing milk. Repeat the cleansing using a cream. Be gentle when removing cleanser.

Normal skin cleansing

Morning Use either a cleansing milk or a balanced cleansing bar.

Evening Remove make-up with cleansing milk, then repeat with milk or a cleansing bar.

Note: Always remove cleansing cream or milk with dampened cotton wool. This glides easily over the skin without dragging and is much kinder than tissues. If you like to use a flannel to remove traces of the cleansing bar, make sure it's scrupulously clean. Flannels and sponges are perfect hosts for harmful bacteria.

Aromatherapy cleansers

Using your favourite unperfumed cleansing cream or milk, add any of the following aromatherapy oils, either singly or in combination for each skin type. The ratio is two drops of oil to every 4 fl oz (100 ml) of cleanser.
Dry skin Camomile, geranium, rose, ylang-ylang
Chapped, cracked skin Benzoin, camomile
Hyper-sensitive skin Camomile, neroli, jasmine, rose
Broken capillaries Neroli, rose, lemon, peppermint
Combination skin Lavender, geranium
Normal skin Rose, neroli, lavender, sandalwood

Balancing

Skin tonics, or fresheners, have two effects on your skin after cleansing.

1. They remove the last trace of cleansing milk or cream.
2. They help to restore the skin's natural protective mantle.

However oily your skin is, I wouldn't recommend you to use a skin tonic containing alcohol (often called an astringent). I find these strip away the skin's natural protective barrier, and with prolonged use can sensitize the skin or cause irritation.

There are lots of commercially available skin tonics and fresheners, but below I've given some ideas for lovely products using beneficial aromatherapy oils. By the way, rosewater and orange flower water can be bought at most good chemists'.

As with the cleansers, the ratio is two drops of

aromatherapy oil to 4 fl oz (100 ml) of toner, either used singly or in combination.

Oily skin

Add lemon, lavender, bergamot, juniper or ylang-ylang to witch hazel.

Acne

Add lemon grass, lavender, juniper or camomile to distilled or mineral water

Dry skin

Add rose, ylang-ylang, geranium or camomile to rosewater.

Hyper-sensitive skin

Add camomile, neroli, jasmine or rose to orange flower water.

Normal skin

Add lavender, rose or neroli, to rosewater or orange flower water.

As with cleansers, all fresheners/toners are kindest when applied to your skin with damp cotton wool. Gently wipe all over the face and neck, paying careful attention to the creases around your chin. If necessary, repeat once more.

Moisturizing

A moisturizer will protect your skin from moisture loss, helping to keep it soft, smooth and supple. It will also protect your skin from the penetration of grime, chemicals and bacteria. We all need moisturizers, even those of us with the most oily skin, but obviously it's important to choose the correct one for your skin type.

Apply moisturizer to your skin while it is still slightly

damp from balancing. This enhances the moisturizing effect. Spread it gently, first on to your neck, then up on to your face, being careful not to drag the skin — particularly around the delicate eye area.

Make sure you use a moisturizer with a vegetable oil base. Mineral oil is not compatible with skin, so baby lotion and petroleum jelly products are therefore best avoided.

Try any of the following to turn your day or night cream into a beneficial aromatherapy treatment.

Again, the ratio is two drops of aromatherapy oil to 4 fl oz (100 ml) of cream, either used singly or in combination.

Oily skin
Day cream Lavender, basil, camomile, lemon
Night cream Lavender, neroli, camomile

Acne
Day cream Lemongrass, bergamot, lavender

Dry skin
Day cream Rose, geranium, neroli
Night cream Frankincense (renowned for its rejuvenating effect), jasmine, rose, ylang-ylang

Hyper-sensitive skin
Day cream Camomile, lavender
Night cream Neroli, jasmine, rose, camomile

Broken capillaries
Day cream Peppermint, lavender, lemon
Night cream Neroli, rose, camomile

Normal skin
Day cream Lavender, rose
Night cream Lavender, rose, neroli

Chapter 5

AROMATHERAPY AND PREGNANCY

The gentle, healing action of aromatherapy is particularly helpful during pregnancy, when it is not advisable to take medication except under the watchful eye of your doctor.

In this chapter you will see how aromatherapy oils can help to lessen the niggly, uncomfortable problems, such as nausea (morning sickness), swollen hands and feet, general aches and pains and fatigue. They can also help you to relax, and look after your body as it slowly goes through changes. Please be sensible, though. If there's anything you're unsure of regarding your health, do check with your doctor first.

IN THE BEGINNING (FIRST TO THIRD MONTHS)

The first three months of pregnancy are the most taxing for your body. During these early stages 'blooming' may be the last thing you feel. Rest is very important, so allow time to relax and wind down before going off to bed. You could also try burning one of the relaxing base note oils in your bedroom, to help you sleep.

You may feel nauseous, particularly between the

eighth and tenth weeks, when one of the pregnancy hormones is at its peak.

Your skin and hair can take a bashing early on in pregnancy when a sudden increase in your hormone levels activates the sebaceous glands, increasing the oiliness of your skin and hair. Luckily, this usually corrects itself during the next few months, but you should be extra scrupulous right now and, if necessary, reassess your skin type.

Fatigue

Try to relax prior to going to bed. Either try a relaxing aromatherapy bath or burn one of the following blends of oil in the room you are in before going off to bed, then take the burner/vaporizer into your bedroom.

☆ Camomile and lavender
☆ Sandalwood
☆ Neroli and ylang-ylang

THE MIDDLE MONTHS (FOURTH TO SIXTH MONTHS)

Nausea, tiredness and irritability should all have lifted by now, and you will probably feel you can take on the world. This is a good time to start making your body more flexible, and to learn relaxation and breathing techniques. Aromatherapy oils are great aids to relaxation, so don't overlook them.

Start to look after your skin (on both your face and body) religiously now. It may seem a chore, but it will pay dividends later. Your weight will have increased quite noticeably already, putting extra strain on your pelvis, back and legs. Varicose veins and spider veins often first appear during pregnancy, so try to take as many preventive measures as possible now. Support tights help, as do regular moderate exercise and the aromatherapy treatment I've suggested.

Constipation can sometimes be a problem in the early stages of pregnancy, but avoid the use of laxatives. Instead, try to eat high-fibre and raw foods and drink plenty of water, or try the aromatherapy remedy in this chapter.

Morning sickness or nausea

If you're feeling nauseous, but not actually vomiting, mix up a blend of two drops each of fennel, lavender and sandalwood oils with 4 fl oz (100 ml) of a carrier oil. Massage it into your abdomen at regular intervals during the day, and try a little dabbed under your nose so you can inhale it. Inhaling peppermint oil can also relieve morning sickness, but I wouldn't advise you to massage with it during pregnancy.

Vomiting

If you're vomiting, mix up a blend of two drops each of lemon, fennel and rose oil with 4 fl oz (100 ml) of a carrier oil. Gently massage it into your upper and lower abdomen, and also inhale it — if you can bear it.

Constipation

Try to relieve your constipation naturally by watching your diet (eat more unrefined food) and increasing your liquid intake. A helpful aromatherapy mixture is three drops of black pepper and three drops of fennel oil in 4 fl oz (100 ml) of a carrier oil. Gently massage it along your lower abdomen, starting just inside your right hip bone, work up, then across past your navel and back down towards your left hip bone, as shown in the illustration. *Be gentle* and repeat several times daily.

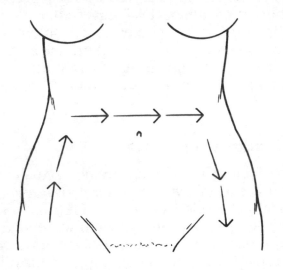

Tired legs/varicose veins

Add three drops of lemon and three drops of lavender oil to 4 fl oz (100 ml) of a light carrier oil, such as grapeseed oil. Massage daily (twice a day, if time allows) from the ankle firmly up to the knee, then firmly up to the top of the thigh. Repeat these movements until the oil is absorbed. After the treatment try to spend at least half an hour with both feet raised above hip level.
Note: Try to avoid very hot baths as they can weaken the capillaries and cause little broken veins under your skin, particularly on your thighs. You are extra vulnerable to these during pregnancy.

THE FINAL MONTHS (SEVEN TO NINE MONTHS)

By now you will be carrying an extra 15 pounds (6.75 kilos) or more in weight. You will probably tire quickly and may even sometimes feel dizzy. Sleep can become a problem as it is difficult to find a comfortable position in bed.

Try lying on your side with a cushion under your uppermost leg, knees slightly bent. The cushion acts as a support and will lessen the strain on your lower back.

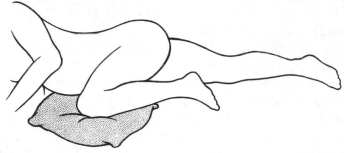

Towards the end of pregnancy a lot of women find their hands and feet swell up, especially during hot weather. Counteract this by drinking plenty of water (to aid kidney function) and trying the appropriate aromatherapy treatment.

Difficulty sleeping

Ask your partner to gently massage your lower back, shoulders and neck with an aromatherapy blend made from three drops of vetivert and three drops of lavender oil in 4 fl oz (100 ml) of a carrier oil. This is a sedative, being calming and relaxing, and it has certainly helped me through some sleepless nights.

You can also try drinking camomile tea before going to bed, and put a little of the above blend on your pillow.

Fluid retention

Mix two drops of eucalyptus oil, two drops of geranium oil and two drops of lavender oil with 4 fl oz (100 ml) of a light carrier oil. Rub it gently into your lower legs and hands. Massage with firm upward strokes — on your legs from ankle to knee, on your arms from hand to elbow. You can also try using the blend in a coolish bath.

Sore nipples

Your breasts will have grown larger throughout pregnancy, and you may have noticed your nipples have darkened and become softer. From the middle months onwards drops of colostrum (the baby's first food if you breast feed) are secreted from your nipples and sometimes they can become sore and cracked.

The following aromatherapy treatment is healing and soothing, and can be continued while you breast feed. Add six drops of marigold oil (often known as calendula) to 4 fl oz (100 ml) of a carrier oil (wheatgerm oil is good). Apply two or three times a day. You can add the marigold oil to a fragrance-free cream, if you prefer.

GENTLE WAYS TO MASSAGE

I've already talked at length about the benefits of massage in Chapter 3. It is an excellent way for you and your partner to get to know the feel of your body, and the way it is changing, throughout pregnancy. Obviously, extra care needs to be taken when working on more vulnerable areas, such as your tummy and lower back, but they can still be worked on, and you will find here some nice, gentle massage movements to try.

During pregnancy, the amount of aromatherapy oil you add to the carrier oil should be reduced by half, because your body is much more sensitive to the oils when you are pregnant, and better able to absorb them. Nevertheless, you will still receive an effective treatment, so don't be tempted to add a few more drops just in case.

This relaxation massage is simple to learn, and you could even give it to a pregnant friend. The lovely aromatherapy scents are also relaxing and help alleviate tension which is often present during pregnancy.

Use the tips in Chapter 3 to create the right aromatherapy atmosphere. Make sure your partner is comfortable, then begin. If your partner is more than four months' pregnant she will find it uncomfortable to lie on her front. Instead, help her to lie on her side supported by a cushion, or massage her back while she is in a sitting position, with a cushion to lean on for support.

Massaging the back

Gently apply your chosen oil to your partner's back, shoulders and arms.

1. Stroke gently down the spine from the base of the neck to the lower back. Do this slowly and evenly and repeat, using alternate hands, twenty times.
2. With both hands, gently stroke down the sides of the neck, over the shoulders and down the arms, coming off at the hands. Repeat ten times.
3. With both hands, stroke gently up the spine, round the shoulder blades in a figure-of-eight, then gently down the sides of the body. Repeat ten times.
4. Stroke across the back, starting from the lower back on the right hand side. Stroke in from the outside of

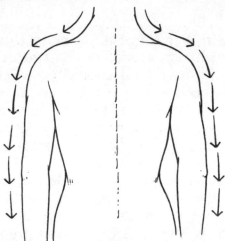

the body towards the spine with alternate hands, moving gently up the back towards the shoulders. Repeat several times on the right side, then work on the left side in the same way.

5. Place one hand on your partner's lower back, place your other hand on top, and allow the heat from your hands to build up. This is very soothing to a sore back.

6. Repeat step 1.

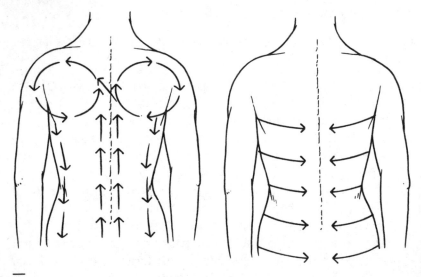

Now work on your partner's neck to ease tension.

1. Knead along from the outer shoulders towards the base of the neck. Repeat four or five times.
2. With your fingertips, work in little circular movements from the base of the neck up to the base of the skull. Repeat four or five times.
3. Stroke down the sides of the neck and out to the shoulders, very slowly. Repeat five or six times.

Now, turn your partner on to her back. (She may like the support of a rolled-up towel under her knees.)

Massaging the tummy

Gently apply your chosen oil to your partner's tummy.

1. Gently stroke down the tummy from between the breasts to the pubic bone. Repeat twenty times with alternate hands.

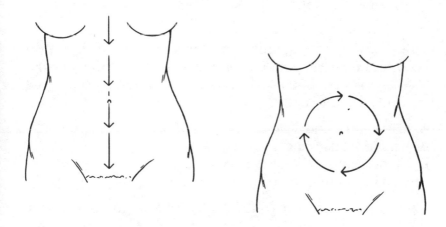

2. Gently circle around the tummy with the flat of your hand in a clockwise direction. Do not apply any pressure. Think of this as a way to soothe and calm your partner. Repeat five or six times.

3. Stroke in from the hip bone, using alternate hands, gradually moving up the body to the side of the chest. Repeat several times on each side.

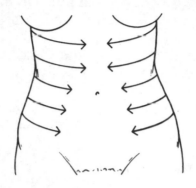

4. This movement is helpful for an aching, tired back. Reach under your partner's waist with both hands. Now slide them out from under her back, lifting gently as you do so. Bring your hands gently over her tummy. Repeat five or six times.
5. Repeat step 1.

This massage is mainly for relaxation, and I would recommend that you try one of the following aromatherapy blends. Use six drops of aromatherapy oil to 4 fl oz (100 ml) of carrier oil.

☆ Camomile and lavender
☆ Frankincense and neroli
☆ Ylang-ylang and sandalwood
☆ Geranium and rose

Alternatively, use any of the above oils singly in a carrier oil.

HELP FOR STRETCH MARKS

Stretch marks are actually little tears in the tissue beneath the skin surface, and they show up first as red or purplish marks which fade to a silvery white scar. They are caused by the skin stretching as your weight increases, and you are more prone to them during pregnancy when your weight gain is rapid. Some skins have a better capacity to stretch than others, so pregnancy doesn't necessarily mean you'll get stretch marks. Although I don't believe that by applying oils and lotions you can prevent stretch marks (the damage occurs quite deep in the skin), you can help to keep your skin elastic and supple. Also, by using aromatherapy oils, you can minimize the scarring and speed up the skin's healing process.

Aromatherapy stretch mark oil

Add three drops of frankincense and three drops of tangerine oil to a carrier blend of 2 fl oz (50 ml) of avocado oil and 2 fl oz (50 ml) of wheatgerm oil. Frankincense has a rejuvenating effect on your skin and tangerine oil is rich in Vitamin C and helps to maintain your skin's elasticity.

I recommend you start using this blend from the beginning of your pregnancy, paying special attention to your breasts, tummy, hips and thighs. Massage it gently into all those areas at least once a day. A good time to do this is at night, after your bath, when your skin is soft.

You may also like to try the following breast massage, as your breasts will increase in size during pregnancy and are therefore prone to stretch marks and tissue damage.

Breast massage

Apply the stretch mark oil to your breasts.

1. Gently work around each breast in a circular movement with your whole hand. Repeat five or six times.
2. Now, place the heel of each hand on either side of one breast and gently stroke in towards the nipple. Repeat five or six times.
3. Next, move your hands to the top and underside of the breast and again stroke in to the nipple. Repeat five or six times.
4. Gently stretch each nipple with your fingertips.
5. Repeat step 1

AROMATHERAPY DURING LABOUR

The experience of labour is different for every woman, as I've found out through treating lots of women through their pregnancies and on after their baby has been born. What they do agree on, however, is the importance of being able to relax, and that the touch of their partner is both reassuring and relieving.

Using aromatherapy massage during labour helps you to relax and cope with the contractions, and it can also reduce the tension and fear you will naturally feel because of its calming effect on your nervous system. You may find that early on in labour you like the feeling of quite firm pressure but as your contractions become more intense gentle strokes may be all you can bear. It's up to you.

If you've already experienced aromatherapy massage earlier in your pregnancy your partner will have an idea of the kind of touch that is most helpful to you.

Tummy massage

This is helpful in the earlier stages of labour, and the movements are soothing when the contractions feel like period pains. Use three drops of camomile or lavender oil in 4 fl oz (100 ml) of a light carrier oil.

1. Using relaxed hands, make a figure-of-eight movement across the tummy and under the 'bump'. This movement should be fairly light, especially if the tummy is tender.
2. Gently stroke around the bump, using your fingertips in a circular movement.

Repeat these movements as necessary.

Back soother

Again, use three drops of camomile or lavender oil in 4 fl oz (100 ml) of a carrier oil.

1. With the heel of your hand apply pressure to the small of the back. Gently move your hand in an anti-clockwise circular movement while keeping firm contact with the skin.
2. Place one hand on top of the other in the small of the back and allow heat to build up under your hands.

These movements are helpful for contractions felt in the lower back.

If you are feeling too sensitive to be massaged or even touched on your body, try the following aromatherapy relaxers.

Face soother

Add a few drops of lavender or rose oil to some chilled rosewater. Dip a small face sponge into this mixture, then smooth it over your forehead, down your face and neck, gently and rhythmically. Alternatively, your partner can do this for you. The flowery aroma is very comforting, and helps to take your mind away from the labour pains.

Scented water soother

Kneeling in a deep, warm bath can be soothing in the earlier stages of labour, and the addition of relaxing aromatherapy oils intensifies this experience. Choose from:

☆ Camomile   ☆ Ylang-ylang
☆ Lavender   ☆ Geranium

Your partner can help take your mind off the pains by rhythmically pouring warm, scented water down your back.

Hand soother

When the contractions become difficult, this simple touch is very reassuring and helps to create a feeling of safety.

1. Ask your partner to rub a little lavender oil (in a carrier oil) into the solar plexus area on your hand.
2. Now, he or she can gently stroke and soothe your hand, keeping a reassuring contact with you. Concentrate on relaxing into the touch.

One for your partner

If he or she is becoming weary, inhaling the following can help. Inhale neat: ☆ Neroli
☆ Rosemary   ☆ Lavender
☆ Petigrain   ☆ Peppermint

Chapter 6

TREATS FOR CHILDREN

In this section I will show how you can introduce the pleasures of aromatherapy to the younger members of your family. Kids love trying out anything new, especially when it's fun and enjoyable, and if it involves good smells then all the better! I've yet to come across a child who hasn't enjoyed an aromatherapy bath using zingy citrus oils in the water.

Baby massage is perhaps unusual in this country, but in the east, and particularly India, it is quite traditional. It may take you a little time to get used to the idea of massaging a wriggling baby, but you'll find he or she will gradually relax and respond to your touch. Massage is a lovely way of strengthening the bond developing between you, too.

When using aromatherapy oils on children, make sure you use only half the normal amount in your chosen carrier. For babies I'd cut this down even further to just two drops in 4 fl oz (100 ml) of carrier oil. Remember, you are working on a much smaller surface area, and too much aromatherapy oil can have a slightly toxic effect.

REMEDIES FOR COMMON CHILDHOOD AILMENTS

Although I'm not suggesting you use aromatherapy to treat your child's measles or tonsillitis (though you can use oils to relieve some of the symptoms) there are many times when aromatherapy can give just the relief your child needs. Problems such as travel sickness, chapped skin, grazes and coughs can all be helped with the choice of the right oil and a little loving administration.

I have found most children like the idea of trying something which isn't a pill or an unpleasant-tasting medicine. Psychologically, this is a good thing because by believing in the treatment they are already on their way to feeling better. And, if they feel better, you feel better!

TRAVEL SICKNESS

Rather than giving travel sickness pills which cause drowsiness, try the following.

Blend six drops of peppermint oil into 4 fl oz (100 ml) of a carrier oil. Massage it into your child's tummy and temples prior to your journey. Also apply a little under his or her nose to inhale. Take the peppermint oil with you so he or she can inhale on the journey, too.

GRAZES

Sometimes grazes can be slow to heal, particularly on knees and elbows where the constant bending pulls the skin. This aromatherapy blend can help.

Firstly clean the graze with ½ pint (300 ml) of warm water, to which you have added four drops of lavender oil. Then, use more lavender oil in a carrier oil (wheatgerm is good for this) to soothe the graze. Repeat the oil application two or three times daily until the graze has healed.

BRUISES

Apply either of the following:

Add three drops of marigold and three drops of camphor oil to a carrier oil. Apply to the bruise several times a day.

Make a compress out of cotton wool soaked in cool water. Apply a couple of drops of neat camphor oil to it and place on the bruise. This will quickly bring out the bruising.

CUTS

Add four drops of tea tree oil to ½ pint (300 ml) of warm water and use it to rinse the cut. Then apply neat tea tree oil to the cut.

NOSE BLEEDS

While your little casualty is sitting forward, pinching his or her nostrils together, make up the following cold compress.

Soak a flannel in 1 pint (600 ml) of very cold water, to which you have added six drops of frankincense oil. Fold it in half and place over the bridge of the nose. Bleeding usually stops very quickly.

TOOTHACHE

The old remedy we are all familiar with — oil of cloves — is just the job, here. It has an anaesthetizing effect on the nerve, lessening pain and bringing a lot of relief until you can get your child to a dentist.

Dip a cotton bud in neat clove oil, then apply to the offending tooth. Repeat as necessary.

For a teething baby, rub the sore gums with a little neat camomile oil several times a day.

MOUTH ULCERS

Mouth ulcers can be a nuisance, and sometimes quite painful. I well remember having a bout of them as a young teenager.

Dip a cotton bud in neat myrrh oil and apply to the ulcer. Repeat as necessary.

Try using this mouthwash as a preventive measure. Add six drops of myrrh oil to a cup of warm water and rinse the mouth out really well. Children usually like this because it involves lots of spitting!

BITES AND STINGS

Dab the bite or sting with neat lavender oil as needed.

SORE THROAT

Either of the following remedies help soothe irritation, or you can use both together if the patient doesn't object. Obviously, very young children can't gargle, so use the oil instead.

To make a mouthwash/gargle, add two drops of lemon, two drops of eucalyptus and two drops of lavender oil to a cup of warm water.

Alternatively, you can add the above oils to 4 fl oz (100 ml) of carrier oil and rub the mixture into the throat and chest, then up into the glands behind the ears, at regular intervals.

ECZEMA

This is a very common childhood complaint and aromatherapy is a very effective way of helping it.

Dry eczema
Add six drops of geranium oil to 4 fl oz (100 ml) of

avocado oil and apply to the affected areas several times daily. You can also add six drops of geranium oil to your child's daily bath.

Weeping eczema
Add six drops of bergamot oil to 4 fl oz (100 ml) of avocado oil and apply to the affected areas several times daily. You can also add six drops of bergamot oil to your child's daily bath.

HICCOUGHS

Children often find hiccoughs a novelty, but they can be irritating and if they don't stop quickly, you can try this.
   Add six drops of fennel oil to 4 fl oz (100 ml) of carrier oil. Rub the mixture along your child's diaphragm, then up his or her chest and throat. You can also allow him or her to inhale neat fennel oil from the bottle (you can use this remedy yourself, increasing the amount of fennel to 12 drops).

TUMMY ACHE

Gentle massage is soothing on its own, but is even more beneficial with the help of aromatherapy.
   Add two drops of camomile, two of fennel and two of peppermint oil to 4 fl oz (100 ml) of carrier oil. Gently rub this into your child's tummy, using soothing massage strokes. Also, try adding the above oils to a warm bath — the heat helps pain and there is no need for a carrier oil.

ASTHMA

If your child suffers from asthma, aromatherapy can help in several ways.
   Add four drops of benzoin and four drops of

rosemary oil to his or her daily bath.

Make up a massage oil using three drops of benzoin and three drops of lavender oil. Rub it into the chest at regular intervals daily.

Also, try using a vaporizer in the child's bedroom at night, with benzoin, pine and rosemary oils (or, any one of them).

COUGHS

Add three drops of eucalyptus and three drops of thyme oil to 4 fl oz (100 ml) of a carrier oil. Massage, or rub, it into your child's chest and throat. These oils are also helpful when inhaled in steam and you can use them in a vaporizer in your child's bedroom at night. Simply place it beside the bed.

BOILS

If you've ever been unfortunate enough to suffer a boil, you'll know how important it is to find some relief.

Make a small compress out of a cotton wool pad and soak it in hot water. Apply neat lemon or myrrh oil to the boil, then cover with the hot pad. Repeat applications regularly to draw the boil.

SUNBURN

However careful you are with protective creams and lotions, sometimes a little patch of skin seems to burn. Instant relief is at hand.

Apply neat lavender oil if the area is small. For larger areas, make up a spray by adding 12 drops of lavender oil to ½ pint (300 ml) of cold water. Spray the affected areas as needed. This is really good for sore skin because it is very soothing and avoids having to touch the affected area.

NAPPY RASH AND SORE CHAFED SKIN

Commercial baby oils are made with mineral oil, which can eventually be drying to delicate skin: sweet almond oil is much kinder. To make an aromatherapy baby oil, add four drops of rose or camomile oil to 4 fl oz (100 ml) of sweet almond oil. This is very soothing when stroked on nappy rash or irritated skin.

CHAPPED SKIN

Because children are always in a hurry, they don't always dry themselves properly. This can lead to chapped, sore skin, especially in winter.

Add six drops of benzoin or myrrh oil to a carrier oil and rub into the affected areas several times daily.

HELPING YOUR CHILD TO SLEEP

Sleep is vital to the health of your child (as it is to everyone). Most children sleep like tops after all the activity of a busy day but there are times when even they can have difficulty sleeping. There are many different reasons for this, and I've listed a few here with the various ways in which aromatherapy can be helpful.

FEAR OF THE DARK

This is very common in children, especially if they have nightmares and wake up in a very dark, silent room. Using an oil burner in the bedroom creates a safe atmosphere, because of its gently glowing light and soothing aroma. You can easily take the oil burner away from home, too, to create the same safe atmosphere in a strange place.

The following oils are all quite sedative and you can experiment until you find a blend that your child really likes.

☆ Camomile ☆ Rose
☆ Benzoin ☆ Sandalwood
☆ Frankincense ☆ Marigold
☆ Neroli ☆ Myrrh
☆ Patchouli ☆ Ylang-ylang
☆ Vetivert ☆ Clary sage

HYPERACTIVITY

If your child is hyperactive, the chances are that you will find he or she has difficulty getting off to sleep. Try the following aromatherapy sequence.

First of all, add ten drops of camomile oil to a three-quarters filled bath. Encourage your child to soak in it (while supervised) for as long as possible. Use toys or games to keep him or her interested, or read a story aloud.

Next, use six drops of camomile oil to 4 fl oz (100 ml) of a carrier oil and massage it into your child's back and shoulders, then the tummy and chest. Do this after drying him or her and while standing, and make the movements as soothing as possible. (You may have to turn this into a game as hyperactive children hate keeping still.)

Finally, use camomile and benzoin oils in a burner or vaporizer in the bedroom. Once your little one is tucked up in bed, try massaging a little of the above blend into his or her forehead with soothing strokes while you read a bedtime story.

EXCITABILITY

Children get really keyed up about certain events,

holidays and Christmas being two that spring immediately to mind. The trouble is that by getting exited and not sleeping properly, the occasions they so look forward to are often marred by their irritability and short tempers — the consequences of lack of sleep.

Try using any of the sedative oils in your child's bath, and also in a vaporizer or burner in his or her bedroom. You can also sprinkle a few drops of camomile or ylang-ylang oil on to the pillow.

FEAR AND ANXIETY

Like adults, children often lose sleep through fear or anxiety. The cause may be an impending test or exam, a trip to the dentist, or one of many other problems.

Helpful oils for this are:

☆ Bergamot ☆ Geranium
☆ Thyme ☆ Camomile
☆ Neroli ☆ Lavender
☆ Marjoram

Again, you can use them in the bath, or in a burner or vaporizer. They can also help when inhaled neat from the bottle. Neroli is very effective when used this way. Note: If your child, or teenager, is facing an impending test or examination, use rosemary in his or her bath and in a burner — it's a great aid to the memory! It can also be inhaled just before the test or exam.

BABY MASSAGE

Babies need touch in order to thrive. Paediatric research has shown that babies born prematurely make much quicker progress when given regular massage.

Massaging your baby will probably come naturally to you — it is just an extension of your need to touch and get as close as possible while you look after all his or her other needs. It strengthens the bonds between you and will soothe and calm you both.

The best time to massage your baby is just after his or her bath, when he or she is not feeling hungry or irritable. Make sure the room is nice and warm, and perhaps perfume it gently with a vaporizer and one of the relaxing aromatherapy oils.

You will find it easiest to work sitting on the floor, legs outstretched with the baby lying on your legs. This means he or she is reassured by the warmth of your skin. Make sure you feel comfortable before you start, and if necessary, prop yourself up with a couple of cushions.

You need to remove any jewellery and warm your hands and the oil prior to massage. Use a blend of 4 fl oz (100 ml) of sweet almond oil to which you have added two drops of any of the following:

☆ Camomile oil   ☆ Lavender oil
☆ Rose oil   ☆ Neroli oil

Now you are ready to begin.

THE MASSAGE

1. Start with your baby lying against your legs on his or her back so he or she can look up at you.
2. Stroke gently down his arms, then his legs, repeating each movement five or six times.
3. Circle round his tummy, using the flat of your hand, in an anti-clockwise direction (this is very calming).
4. Stretch out his toes one by one, then gently rub over the soles of his feet, using your thumb.
5. Uncurl his fingers, then gently move each one clockwise, then anti-clockwise. Now, rub over the palms of his hands with your thumb.

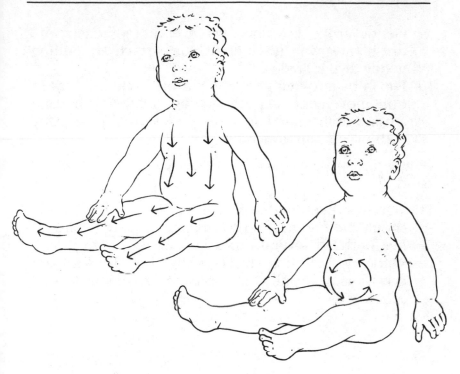

Turn your baby over, to lie on his tummy against your legs.

6. Gently rub a little oil into his back, bottom, legs and feet using long, light strokes.
7. Stroke down his back, giving a little squeeze at the buttocks. Repeat five or six times.
8. Gently stroke round his shoulders, down his arms and off at his hands.

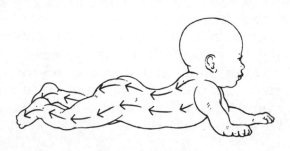

9. Gently stroke down his legs several times. Each time finish by giving his legs a little stretch by pulling gently at the ankles.
10. Finish by stroking gently down his back and legs in one movement. Repeat, getting lighter with each stroke, until your hand just glides over your baby without actually touching him.

Gently turn your baby on to his back so he can see you again.

11. Gently stroke a little oil (the surplus on your hands should be enough) on to his face. Lightly stroke up his forehead several times.
12. With your thumbs stroke across his cheeks, then down his nose and chin. Do each movement several times.

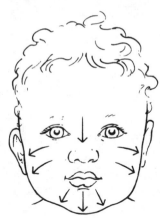

13. Gently squeeze and rub his ear lobes between your finger and thumb.
14. Finish off with a connecting stroke. With one hand cradling your baby's head, stroke gently down his body with the other and bring it to rest on top of his feet. Hold this position (one hand on the head, the other on the feet) for a count of ten. Gently release and lift off your hands.

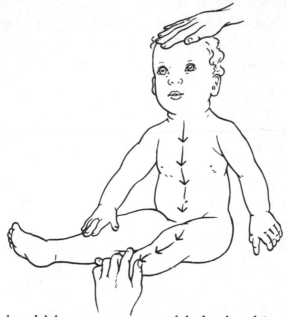

You should have a contented baby by this point!

AROMATHERAPY FOR YOUR BABY

As well as massage, there are other ways in which you can treat your baby to aromatherapy. Just be careful to keep the amount of aromatherapy oil very low, as this is enough for a baby or young child.

As a guide use:

☆ Two drops of aromatherapy oil in 4-6 fl oz (100-150 ml) of a carrier oil, or two to four drops of aromatherapy oil in a baby bath. The most suitable oils for your baby are the most gentle ones:

☆ Camomile   ☆ Neroli
☆ Lavender   ☆ Sandalwood
☆ Rose   ☆ Tangerine

The best carrier oil for babies is sweet almond oil, as it has a softening, lubricating effect on the skin and is much kinder than the mineral oil that most commercial baby products are based on.

BABY BATH

Most babies enjoy being immersed in water (after all, they spent nine months floating in amniotic fluid) and you can add soothing aromatherapy oils to their baths to create a lovely smell, and soothe their sensitive skins. Camomile, rose or lavender oils are best for this and are much kinder than proprietary baby bubble baths.

THE NURSERY

Try using any of the following oils in a vaporizer in your baby's room. They help to purify the air and keep germs at bay as well as being pleasant and soothing.

☆ Lavender   ☆ Camomile
☆ Frankincense   ☆ Eucalyptus
☆ Sandalwood   ☆ Geranium
☆ Neroli

If your baby has been having disturbed sleep, try popping a little ball of cotton wool, to which you've added a couple of drops of camomile oil, far inside his pillowcase. He'll breathe in its soothing vapours as he sleeps.

TEETHING

When your baby is teething, camomile oil helps to calm and soothe inflamed gums. Dilute two drops in a little warm water and rub over the affected area three times a day.

CRADLE CAP

This flaky, red, itchy condition often affects small babies. You can ease it with aromatherapy.

Mix up a blend of one drop of camomile oil and one drop of rose oil in 4 fl oz (100 ml) of sweet almond oil. Gently rub over the cradle cap three times a day.

You can add two drops of camomile oil to your baby's shampoo, but be careful to rinse his hair thoroughly after shampooing. All shampoos can irritate a sensitive skin.

COLDS AND BLOCKED NOSES

When your baby has a stuffy nose or a cold, use any of the following oils in a vaporizer. They eliminate germs, and help to ease breathing.

☆ Lavender   ☆ Lemon
☆ Eucalyptus   ☆ Pine
☆ Thyme   ☆ Rosemary

Chapter 7

AROMATHERAPY FOR EVERYONE

Aromatherapy is not just a beauty treatment but is also a gentle way of helping to restore the body's natural resilience to viruses, infections and fatigue. In addition, it is particularly helpful for stress-related conditions, so men can gain just as much benefit from it as women.

In this chapter you will find many aromatherapy treatments for all sorts of ailments and stress-related problems that can afflict both sexes. There are also treatments to be used before and after sport or vigorous exercise, plus a few ideas on how to recover when you've over-indulged in food and drink!

HELP FOR STRESS

First of all, let's look at some of the most common symptoms of stress, both physical and emotional.

Physical signs
☆ Pain/tension in the back, neck and shoulders
☆ Headache/migraine
☆ Constipation
☆ General aches and pains
☆ Fatigue/excessive tiredness
☆ Insomnia

Emotional signs
☆ Anxiety
☆ Depression
☆ Irritability/lack of concentration
☆ Lack of confidence
☆ Aggressiveness

When feeling the effects of stress, we tend to use props, which give us a quick lift or calm us down. These can be:

☆ Alcohol
☆ Tea or coffee
☆ Cigarettes/cigars
☆ Chocolate

☆ Excessive eating
☆ Anti-depressants
☆ Sleeping pills

Some stress can be productive: it can give you drive and energy, and help you to achieve goals, but too much is detrimental. A healthy attitude to stress is to recognize it and try to reduce its effect on your health and well-being. This is where you can turn to the gentle healing of aromatherapy. Because the emotional symptoms lead to the physical ones, it is always best to treat them first. Often, then, the physical symptoms won't develop!

Anxiety

These oils can help you:

☆ Lavender
☆ Clary sage
☆ Neroli

☆ Jasmine
☆ Marigold
☆ Vetivert

You can add up to ten drops of whichever oil you think smells best to your bath, then soak in it for at least 15 minutes.
Or inhale neat oil.
Or make up a blend, using up to 12 drops of oil in 4 fl oz (100 ml) of a carrier oil. Massage it into your solar

plexus (just between your ribs) in an anti-clockwise direction. This is very calming.

I find a blend of equal parts of lavender and vetivert oils very good.

DEPRESSION

These oils can help you:

☆ Clary sage
☆ Marjoram
☆ Camomile
☆ Sandalwood

☆ Lavender
☆ Frankincense
☆ Ylang-ylang

You can use them in the bath — up to ten drops in a full tub.
Or inhale them neat, or use in a burner or vaporizer.
Or add 12 drops to 4 fl oz (100 ml) of a carrier oil for massage.

A blend of lavender, clary sage and camomile is good for massage.

Irritability/lack of concentration

These oils can help you:

☆ Camomile
☆ Lavender
☆ Marjoram

☆ Neroli
☆ Rose
☆ Vetivert
☆ Rosemary

You can use them in the bath.
Or use them for steam inhalation.
Or inhale them neat (particularly rosemary and neroli) for quick relief.
Or use them in a burner or vaporizer.

Lack of confidence

These oils can help you:
* ☆ Rosemary
* ☆ Neroli
* ☆ Petitgrain
* ☆ Jasmine

You can inhale them neat for a quick uplift.
Or use them in your bath.
Or use them in a burner or vaporizer.

Aggressiveness

These oils can help you:

* ☆ Lemon
* ☆ Camomile
* ☆ Juniper
* ☆ Marjoram
* ☆ Ylang-ylang

You can use 12 drops in 4 fl oz (100 ml) of a carrier oil for massage, concentrating on the solar plexus and abdomen. A nice blend is lemon, marjoram and ylang-ylang.
Or use them in your bath.

Pain/muscle tension

These oils can help you:

* ☆ Eucalyptus
* ☆ Juniper
* ☆ Black pepper
* ☆ Lavender
* ☆ Rosemary

The best way to treat pain and tension is with massage. Get your partner to work on your back, neck and shoulders with one of the above oils in a carrier oil, or try a little self-massage (see Chapter 3).

I find that eucalyptus is a great pain-reliever. For maximum benefit, use it in the bath, then follow with an aromatherapy massage.

Fatigue/excessive tiredness

These oils can help you:

☆ Lavender
☆ Neroli
☆ Juniper

☆ Rosemary
☆ Geranium

You can use up to ten drops in your bath and soak in it for five to ten minutes.
Or use six drops in a footbath if you're in a hurry.
Or add six drops to 2 fl oz (50 ml) of a carrier oil. Rub it briskly into your solar plexus to uplift and boost energy levels.

Insomnia

These oils can help you:

☆ Camomile
☆ Sandalwood
☆ Ylang-ylang

☆ Patchouli
☆ Neroli
☆ Marjoram

You can use ten drops in your bath and soak well.
Or for massage use 12 drops in 4 fl oz (100 ml) of a carrier oil.
Or inhale neat and sprinkle a few drops on your pillow.

Camomile is one of the most sedative oils and you could also try using it in a burner, and drinking camomile tea before you go to bed.

TREATMENTS FOR SKIN, HAIR AND BODY

Here are simple ways in which aromatherapy can help you take better care of yourself.

Shaving rash

Often called razor burn, this can be anything from dry flaky skin, to really red, sore irritation after shaving. Shaving flakes off dead cells from the skin's surface, therefore leaving your skin extra-sensitive. Aftershaves usually contain alcohol, and can irritate an already sensitive skin.

Add three drops of clary sage oil and three drops of lavender to ½ pint (300 ml) of rosewater or orange flower water. Pat on your face after shaving and repeat two to three hours later.

Athlete's foot

This is a common problem which certainly doesn't only affect athletes! It's caused by a fungus that loves dark, moist areas of skin, hence its favourite breeding ground between the toes.

It is important to wash and dry your feet thoroughly each day, and the following aromatherapy treatment is really good.

Add ten drops of tea tree oil to a footbath of warm water. Soak your feet in it for fifteen to thirty minutes. Repeat daily until the condition begins to improve, then weekly after that.

Dandruff

This scalp disorder seems to affect nearly everyone at some time in their lives. It occurs when dead skin cells accumulate on the scalp and fail to shed themselves normally. They build up, then fall off in large scales. There are other problems which have similar symptoms to dandruff, such as psoriasis and eczema, so if in any doubt check with your doctor.

Try massaging the following blend into your scalp twice a week before shampooing. Leave on for thirty minutes before washing with a mild shampoo. Add six drops of rosemary and four drops of cedarwood oil to 4 fl oz (100 ml) of jojoba or avocado oil. Also add one drop of each essential oil to your final rinsing water after shampooing.

Hay fever

This is actually an allergic reaction caused by the pollens of various shrubs, trees and grasses. Symptoms include sneezing, running nose and sore red eyes. Aromatherapy can ease hay fever, but won't cure it.

Add six drops of hyssop oil to a bowl of hot water and inhale the steam. Alternatively, mix six drops of hyssop oil in 2 fl oz (50 ml) of a carrier oil and massage it into your cheeks and under your nose regularly.
Important note: People prone to epilepsy should avoid hyssop.

Jet lag

This affects you when your internal body clock becomes disorientated. It can cause changes in your normal eating and sleep patterns and is generally debilitating.

During your flight (if it is long haul) drink plenty of water and soft drinks, avoid alcohol and eat little. Sleep, if you can, and before travelling, make up this aromatherapy blend. Add four drops of rosemary, four drops of ylang-ylang and four drops of lemon oil to 4 fl oz (100 ml) of a carrier oil. During your flight, massage it into your neck, face and the back of your neck up to the base of your skull. On arrival, pour some of the blend into a warm bath and soak in it for at least 15 minutes.

Headache/migraine

These oils can help:

☆ Lavender   ☆ Camomile
☆ Peppermint   ☆ Rosemary

You can add 12 drops of oil to 4 fl oz (100 ml) of a carrier oil and massage it into your temples, neck and up into the base of your skull and scalp. If you do this early enough you can prevent the onset of a full-blown headache.

Or steam inhale, using twenty drops of oil in 2 pints (1.1 litres) of hot water. If you have nausea with your headache, peppermint is really helpful.

Constipation

These oils can help:

☆ Rosemary   ☆ Black pepper
☆ Juniper   ☆ Fennel

You can add 12 drops of oil to 4 fl oz (100 ml) of a carrier oil and massage it into your abdomen (see Chapter 5).

Or add twenty drops to your bath and soak in it for fifteen minutes.

General aches and pains

These oils can help:

☆ Eucalyptus   ☆ Rosemary
☆ Black pepper   ☆ Camomile

You can use up to ten drops in your bathwater and soak in it.

Or ask your partner to massage the affected area.

Or try self-massage.

Sunburn

I feel really strongly that prevention is the best cure for this, but if you do burn apply neat lavender oil to soothe the area and prevent infection. Repeat the application every few minutes until the pain lessens.

SPORT

Preparation

Warming up before any strenuous activity is important if you are not to over-stretch or strain your body. Below I've listed some warming oils which I suggest you mix into a carrier oil and rub well into your legs, arms, shoulders and lower back at least 15 minutes before your exercise session.

☆ Benzoin   ☆ Clary sage   ☆ Ginger
☆ Black pepper   ☆ Clove   ☆ Marjoram
☆ Cajaput

Aftercare

After vigorous exercise your muscles cool down and the fibres start to shorten again. This can cause aches and pains, and the joints become stiff. Speed up your recovery with the following relaxing oils:

☆ Benzoin   ☆ Jasmine   ☆ Sandalwood
☆ Camomile   ☆ Lavender   ☆ Vetivert
☆ Frankincense

You can add one to your bath and soak for at least 15 minutes.

Or mix into a carrier oil and use for self-massage (see Chapter 3).

Or ask a friend or partner to massage aching areas.

Here are a couple of specific blends to help.

Aches and pains/sprains

Add ten drops of juniper, ten drops of rosemary and five drops of lemongrass oil to 6 fl oz (150 ml) of a carrier oil.

Cramp

Add ten drops of juniper, ten drops of marjoram and five drops of lemongrass to 6 fl oz (150 ml) of a carrier oil. It's a good idea to massage this into your calf muscles after sport to ward off an attack of cramp.

OVER-INDULGENCE AIDS

Hangover

The morning-after feeling is one we all know, and dread. The prime cause of a hangover (headache, upset stomach, lethargy, nausea) is dehydration, so try to drink plenty of water (or fruit juice, if your stomach can stand it) on waking — and last thing the night before, if possible. Then try the following aromatherapy treatment.

First, make a cold compress to which you add one drop of juniper oil and one drop of fennel oil. Apply to your forehead and temples. Next, blend three drops of rose oil in 1 fl oz (25 ml) of a carrier oil and massage it into the liver area — the lower right side of your ribs and just below them.

Rose oil helps to detoxify the liver. Drinking plenty of water throughout the day is important as well as it will flush the toxins out of your system more efficiently.

Indigestion

This is a horrible acid feeling in your stomach, often experienced after a rich or heavy meal. Help is at hand in the form of peppermint oil, which is a great remedy for digestive problems.

Add 12 drops of peppermint oil to 4 fl oz (100 ml) of a carrier oil and gently massage it into your stomach and solar plexus. Also, dab a little of the blend under your nose so you can inhale it. If you wish, you can follow the treatment with a cup of mint tea.

Chapter 8

QUESTIONS AND ANSWERS

Here are some of the questions I am most frequently asked when working as an aromatherapist. I hope you'll find the answers helpful!

What is aromatherapy?

It is a complimentary therapy — that is, a gentle way of helping to restore the body and mind to a balanced, healthy state, using healing essences extracted from plants, shrubs and trees.

In aromatherapy these are usually applied to the body by way of a gentle massage, although they can be used effectively in other ways. Apart from their healing powers (which include being antiseptic and anti-inflammatory), these aromatherapy plant essences exude powerful scents which have an effect on the memory and sensory nerves. As a result, aromatherapy treats the whole person, both mind and body. It is a very helpful way of treating the stress-related problems that many of us seem to suffer now that our lives have become so pressured.

Does it work for everyone?

Aromatherapy, correctly used, helps us to keep healthy by improving the circulation, soothing the nervous system, reducing waste products and lessening the effects of stress. It can also be used to help chronic conditions such as migraine, eczema, rheumatism and sinus problems, offering more relief to some sufferers than others.

Obviously, there are acute conditions which you wouldn't treat with aromatherapy, such as heart attacks and appendicitis. These need immediate medical attention, not aromatherapy which, I think, is most helpful to stress-related problems. Always remember that if you are in any doubt about a health problem, do consult your doctor before trying to treat the problem yourself.

What happens the first time I have a professional aromatherapy treatment?

You are given a consultation before treatment begins. This is important as it gives the aromatherapist a clearer picture of you and the problem for which you need help.

You will be asked your:
☆ Name
☆ Address
☆ Date of birth
☆ Occupation
☆ Doctor's name and address

Then you will be asked about your:
☆ Medical history — any serious illnesses or operations
☆ General health
☆ Diet and whether you smoke or drink alcohol
☆ Present medication
☆ Exercise
☆ Allergies

You will be encouraged to mention any emotional problems, worries and stresses in your life, but don't feel obliged to talk about anything you would rather keep to yourself. The aromatherapist will be understanding — he or she is there to help you. If the aromatherapist is sure there is no reason for you not to receive treatment, he will then mix up suitable oils for you.

Once these oils are mixed you will be asked to smell them to ensure you like their aroma. Obviously, you won't derive full benefit from being massaged for an hour or more with an oil you find smells unpleasant.

You will then be asked to undress (usually down to your pants) and helped on to a massage couch. Aromatherapists are used to dealing with shyness, and you will be surprised at how quickly you feel at ease. Only the area of your body being worked on will be exposed. The rest of you will be covered by towels, or a blanket, and kept warm. Usually, the room will have soft lighting and your aromatherapist may play soft background music to help you relax.

As he massages you, your aromatherapist will find areas of tension and congestion. These will be pointed out to you, and you may find these spots a little tender when they are touched. Mostly, though, the massage is extremely soothing and relaxing, and very often you will doze off!

At the end of your massage, which usually takes just over an hour, you may be given a glass of water to drink. This helps to refresh you, and will also flush away some of the toxins which have been released into your system during the massage. You will be allowed to relax for a few minutes while your aromatherapist writes any additional remarks on your record card.

He will then help you to dress, before finally recommending any home treatment (such as baths or inhalations) and perhaps giving you a blend of oils to use between treatments. Also, he will say when he feels other treatments will be beneficial.

How will I feel afterwards?

The feeling after an aromatherapy treatment varies between one person to the next. Most people feel very relaxed, and even a little light-headed, with a sort of floating sensation. Some people find they have a sudden spurt of energy, while others are slightly lethargic after treatment.

I always recommend that you try to relax as much as possible after a session. It is therefore a good idea to book your appointment for the end of the day, rather than during the lunch break of a hectic work schedule, and allow yourself plenty of time to recover afterwards.

Very occasionally, someone's condition may seem to worsen slightly after treatment, but it usually improves within a couple of days.

How often should I be treated?

Your aromatherapist will be your guide. Usually, to start with, treatments are given weekly, then as your condition improves they are reduced to monthly or two-monthly sessions.

If you have a chronic condition, you may continue to receive treatment indefinitely, but once your problem has improved you may feel that you'll just have an occasional treatment if you want to relax. Remember, aromatherapy can be used just to maintain good health and well-being.

Is there any time when I can't have aromatherapy?

Again, your aromatherapist will advise you, but here is a general guide to when treatment is best avoided:

Avoided altogether
☆ When you have a fever or abnormal temperature

☆ Just after a heavy meal
☆ On an empty stomach (if you haven't eaten for six hours)
☆ During the first two days of your period
☆ If you are being treated by your doctor, unless his or her permission has been given.
☆ If you are extremely tired

Avoid local areas
☆ Of recent scar tissue
☆ If any infection, bruising or inflammation is present
☆ If skin is cut or broken
☆ If there has been a recent break or fracture of a bone

The rest of your body can still be treated, but the problem area will be avoided. If you must avoid treatment altogether, you can still use aromatherapy oils in a vaporizer or burner to help you feel better.

Are there any aromatherapy oils I should avoid when buying them for use at home?

Here I've compiled a list of oils I wouldn't consider safe for home use, because they can produce side effects. Instead, they should only be used by trained aromatherapists.

☆ Bitter almond
☆ Origanum
☆ Pennyroyal
☆ Sage
☆ Cassia
☆ Bitter fennel
☆ Cinnamon bark — except in a burner or vaporizer
☆ Savory
☆ Tansy

☆ Mustard
☆ Wintergreen
☆ Rue

Which oils are safe, with proper use?

All of the following oils are safe if used with care.

☆ Benzoin
☆ Bergamot
☆ Black pepper
☆ Clary sage
☆ Camomile
☆ Sweet fennel
☆ Frankincense
☆ Jasmine
☆ Lavender
☆ Ginger
☆ Marjoram
☆ Geranium
☆ Eucalyptus
☆ Grapefruit
☆ Tea tree
☆ Lemongrass

If in doubt about any oil, check with a qualified aromatherapist.

I like the idea of keeping a few aromatherapy oils at home, but I don't want to spend too much money. Which would you recommend?

Here are four oils I wouldn't be without:
Lavender This is one of the most versatile aromatherapy oils of all and is even safe to use neat on the skin. It helps all sorts of problems, from burns to headaches, is great for relieving tension and is naturally antiseptic and

soothing. Buy this one first!

Eucalyptus This is a very helpful oil for all respiratory problems — coughs, colds, catarrh and flu. If used in a vaporizer or burner it keeps germs at bay, so can protect other members of your family from common viruses.

Camomile This is a calming, soothing oil. It is helpful for itchy rashes and dry skin conditions, and because it is sedative, it is useful for encouraging sleep and relaxation.

Tea tree This is a fantastic antiseptic and anti-fungal treatment. Use it to clean up cuts and grazes and to treat such irritating problems as thrush and athlete's foot.

I seem to be allergic to most perfumes. Are aromatherapy oils a suitable alternative?

You may well have an allergic reaction to one of the chemicals that go into the manufacture of perfume. The perfume industry copies chemically the scents of aromatherapy oils, and these sometimes have an irritant effect upon the skin. Aromatherapy oils are natural plant oils, and are generally gentler than chemical perfumes. However, I would recommend that you carry out a patch test, using your chosen blend, before using aromatherapy oils as perfume. It is not unknown to be allergic to them.

Patch test
1. Dab a couple of drops of your chosen aromatherapy blend (not neat oil, unless it is lavender) on to your wrist, or behind your ear if you don't want your reaction to be obvious to others.
2. Wait for 24 hours. If your skin shows any redness, itching or irritation, you should avoid the oils. Perhaps you could try a different blend?

How do I use aromatherapy oils as perfume?

Below, I've listed the most pleasant-smelling aroma-therapy oils under different headings. Perfume is a very personal matter so you will need to experiment to find one you really like.

Remember, you must mix your chosen oil, or oils, into the right carrier oil — ten drops to 4 fl oz (100 ml) is a good amount. I find sweet almond oil is a good carrier, as it seems to hold the perfume.

FLORAL	*ORIENTAL*	*FRESH*
☆ Rose	☆ Ylang-ylang	☆ Petigrain
☆ Neroli	☆ Ginger	☆ Lemon
☆ Jasmine	☆ Frankincense	☆ Tangerine
☆ Geranium	☆ Vetivert	☆ Bergamot
☆ Lavender	☆ Sandalwood	☆ Grapefruit

You can also make your own toilet water by adding any of the above oils to rosewater or orange flower water (ten drops to ½ pint [300 ml]). This gives a lighter, fresher, fragrance but it isn't as long-lasting on your skin.

Can I take the oils internally?

I would not recommend anyone to take essential oils internally. Although it is common practice in France (where aromatherapists use the treatment in this way) I think it is quite hazardous to use aromatherapy oils orally. They work efficiently enough when applied to the skin to make oral use unnecessary.

How often can I use aromatherapy at home?

Because of their gentle way of healing, you can use aromatherapy oils every day. You may choose to use them in your bath one day, for massage another, and in a vaporizer the next. In fact, if you do buy an oil burner or vaporizer, I'd be surprised if you didn't use it everyday.

Obviously, if you suddenly find you have an adverse reaction to an aromatherapy oil, you should stop using it immediately and try a different one instead.

Is it possible to use aromatherapy oils in cooking?

Although it is possible to use some of the herbal essences — e.g. marjoram or thyme — in cooking, it is not something I would advise, because it is difficult to know the dosage you will ingest when eating the food. Use the fresh herb equivalent instead.

Are there aromatherapy oils that might help me when I am dieting?

This question is often asked. I think we are all looking for a magical weight loss formula, but sadly it doesn't exist in aromatherapy. However, you can use the oils to look after your body as you begin to lose weight.

For fluid retention
Add geranium, fennel and juniper oils to your bath.

For cellulite
This is the lumpy fat that collects on your bottom and thighs and has the appearance of orange peel. Make a blend of four drops of juniper, four drops of fennel and four drops of lemon oils in 4 fl oz (100 ml) of a carrier oil. Massage this into the affected areas daily after your bath, when the skin is warm and receptive.

Are there any oils which don't smell too feminine? I'd like to give a massage to my husband/boyfriend

Men prefer either the more woody oils or the citrus ones. Try any of the following:

☆ Vetivert   ☆ Marjoram   ☆ Tangerine
☆ Cedarwood   ☆ Bergamot   ☆ Eucalyptus
☆ Sandalwood   ☆ Lemon
☆ Clary sage   ☆ Lemongrass

Where is the best place to store my aromatherapy oils and for how long will they keep?

As I previously explained, aromatherapy oils are affected by light and heat. They need to be kept in a dark, cool place, preferably in tinted glass bottles. Because the oils evaporate very quickly when neat, you must ensure the tops are firmly screwed on your bottles. It's a good idea to keep them all together in a small box and store it in a cool cupboard.

The oils will keep for about two years if kept properly and the bottles haven't been opened. Once opened, I would aim to use them within six months (label and date the bottle when you first open it).

Are there any oils to be avoided during pregnancy?

Obviously, you should avoid any of the oils I've listed as being unsafe. During pregnancy your body is more sensitive and vulnerable than usual, so it's a good idea to avoid the following oils until your baby is born:

☆ Hyssop
☆ Marjoram
☆ Myrrh

The gentlest oils for use during pregnancy
- ☆ Lavender ☆ Camomile
- ☆ Rose ☆ Jasmine
- ☆ Neroli ☆ Frankincense
- ☆ Tangerine ☆ Ylang-ylang

Always use them at half strength.

Which oils would you recommend I take on holiday abroad for all the family?

Aromatherapy oils can be very useful in different ways when visiting a warmer climate. Here are a few recommendations from personal experience.

Insect repellant
Add ten drops of geranium and ten drops of eucalyptus oil to 4 fl oz (100 ml) of a carrier oil. Dab on to areas likely to be bitten (ankles seem to be favourites with mosquitoes). You can also burn the oils neat in your room at night, to ward off biting insects.

Insect bites and stings
If you are unfortunate enough to be stung or bitten, try rubbing neat lavender oil into the affected area. Re-apply every few minutes until the pain/itching stops.

Sunburn
Lavender is excellent for treating any kind of burn, with sunburn being no exception.

If the burned area is small, apply the oil neat and repeat as necessary. If the area is large, add twenty drops to a cool bath and soak for ten to twenty minutes. You can make a soothing spray (burned skin is so tender when touched) by adding ten drops of lavender oil to 1 pint (300 ml) of cool, clean water. (Mineral water is ideal.) Alternatively, you can add a few drops of lavender oil to your aftersun lotion to speed up the healing process.

Dry/cracked lips

The sun seems to cause this problem just as much as harsh winter weather. Make up a carrier oil of 2 fl oz (50 ml) apricot kernel oil and 2 fl oz (50 ml) of avocado oil. Add six drops of sandalwood and six drops of rose oil. Rub this in to the lips, repeating the application regularly.

Small cuts

Even on holiday, accidents happen. Either apply neat lavender or tea tree oil to the cut. These are both antiseptic and don't sting.

Sunstroke

I once suffered sunstroke as a child in Greece, and remember living on water and cucumber for a week! Sunstroke is the result of severe dehydration, and the resulting symptoms are very like those of a hangover.

Keep the sufferer in a darkened, cool room. One good remedy is to add four drops of juniper, four drops of fennel and four drops of peppermint oil to a coolish bath. Soak for fifteen minutes. Then, rub a little neat lavender oil into his or her temples at regular intervals. The bath helps to reduce his temperature and the lavender oil helps his headache.

Make sure your patient keeps topping up his liquid level with plenty of water (not too cold).

Vomiting/diarrhoea

Due to changes in climate, water and diet, upset stomachs often occur on holiday. Aromatherapy can help.

Vomiting
Add four drops of lemon, four drops of fennel and four drops of peppermint to 4 fl oz (100 ml) of a carrier oil. Massage into the abdomen and solar plexus as needed.

Diarrhoea
Add six drops of lavender, three drops of neroli and three drops of lavender oil to 4 fl oz (100 ml) of a carrier oil. Very gently rub into the lower abdomen and solar plexus areas.

You can also try adding the above oils to a bath to ease stomach cramps.

In winter I seem to suffer from the cold more than other people. Can aromatherapy help?

I, too, seem to feel the cold and am much more relaxed in warmer weather. However, I have found aromatherapy helpful in a number of ways. It is very effective in improving the circulation and this lessens the effect of cold on your body. Massage is useful too. It improves the flow of blood to the skin, warming the surrounding tissues.

Some winter-warming oils are:
☆ Black pepper
☆ Benzoin
☆ Ginger
☆ Clary sage
☆ Marjoram

Use any of them in your bath, and in a carrier oil for massage, on a daily basis.

Chilblains
These are of the one of the hazards of winter weather and occur when your body's temperature control system

closes down too quickly. The capillaries close to your skin's surface constrict, impairing the flow of blood to your feet, and particularly your toes.

For an effective cure, add a few drops of lemon oil to some calendula cream (made from marigold extract and available from your chemist). Rub into the affected area regularly, massaging until the skin feels warm. You can also use lemon oil in a footbath, but don't make it too hot. Remember, extremes of temperature, whether hot or cold, will make chilblains worse.

I've been told aromatherapy can really help depression. Is this true?

Depression has many forms, all of which must be treated seriously. It is divided into four different categories.

Reactive depression This relates to a loss of some kind, such as a death, end of a relationship or redundancy.
Hormone-related depression This can be caused by pregnancy, the menopause or menstrual problems.
Ongoing depression There is no clear cause for this.
Severe depression This may relate to more serious orders, such as schizophrenia.

There is more publicity now about the danger of the prolonged use of tranquillizers which are often prescribed to help relieve depression, so aromatherapy is a gentle and helpful alternative treatment and can be used to balance the nervous system.

Massage is beneficial, too, in calming and soothing ragged nerves and bringing you back in touch with your body. It teaches you how to let go and relax, which is sometimes difficult when you feel depressed.

I would like to point out here that it is important you talk to a medically qualified practitioner about your depression before seeking the help of an aromatherapist, and tell him or her that you are thinking of making an appointment.

Here is a list of some of the oils you can add to your bath to help relieve depression.

- ☆ Bergamot
- ☆ Clary sage
- ☆ Camomile
- ☆ Geranium
- ☆ Lavender
- ☆ Frankincense
- ☆ Jasmine
- ☆ Neroli
- ☆ Patchouli
- ☆ Rose
- ☆ Sandalwood
- ☆ Ylang-ylang

I'm getting married soon and I know I'll be extremely edgy. Is there any way aromatherapy can help?

I have been asked this so many times! Brides always seem to become edge long before their wedding day, losing weight and sleep. Try any of the relaxing oils listed below in the bath, and if you get very tense then treat yourself to a professional aromatherapy massage or two.

- ☆ Benzoin
- ☆ Camomile
- ☆ Neroli
- ☆ Petigrain
- ☆ Clary sage
- ☆ Frankincense
- ☆ Patchouli
- ☆ Sandalwood
- ☆ Geranium
- ☆ Lavender
- ☆ Rose
- ☆ Vetivert

On the morning of your wedding have a relaxing aromatherapy bath, and dab one of the uplifting oils, such as tangerine, under your nose. Massage lavender or rose oil up into the back of your neck and base of your skull to ease tension and ward off nervous headache. You should then be all set for a marvellous day!

INDEX

V